Houseplants for a Healthy Home

50 Indoor Plants to Help You Breathe Better, Sleep Better, and Feel Better All Year Round

Jon VanZile

Adams Media

New York   London   Toronto   Sydney   New Delhi

Adams media

Adams Media
An Imprint of Simon & Schuster, Inc.
57 Littlefield Street
Avon, Massachusetts 02322

First Adams Media hardcover edition May 2018

ADAMS MEDIA and colophon are trademarks of Simon & Schuster.

For information about special discounts for bulk purchases, please contact Simon & Schuster Special Sales at 1-866-506-1949 or business@simonandschuster.com.

The Simon & Schuster Speakers Bureau can bring authors to your live event. For more information or to book an event contact the Simon & Schuster Speakers Bureau at 1-866-248-3049 or visit our website at www.simonspeakers.com.

Interior design by Colleen Cunningham and Katrina Machado
Interior illustrations by Nicola DosSantos

Manufactured in the United States of America

4 2021

Library of Congress Cataloging-in-Publication Data
VanZile, Jon, author.
Houseplants for a healthy home / Jon VanZile.
Avon, Massachusetts: Adams Media, 2018.
LCCN 2017057173 (print) | LCCN 2017058876 (ebook) | ISBN 9781507207291 (hc) | ISBN 9781507207307 (ebook)
LCSH: House plants.
LCC SB419 (ebook) | LCC SB419 .V37 2018 (print) | DDC 635.9/65--dc23
LC record available at https://lccn.loc.gov/2017057173

ISBN 978-1-5072-0729-1
ISBN 978-1-5072-0730-7 (ebook)

Dedication

Always for Erika.

Contents

Acknowledgments

This book was great fun to write, so thanks to everyone who made it possible.

My family—Erika, Max, and Jake—thank you for tolerating long hours at a keyboard. And, Erika, especially, thank you. Every time I might have turned away from pursuing writing as a career, you encouraged me and supported me in sticking with it. I get to live my dream because of you. Thanks also to Jackie Musser, senior editor at Adams Media, for giving me the opportunity to write this book.

And finally, thanks to everyone who has participated in my lifelong education and love of growing things! May your soil always be rich, your blooms profuse, and your water sweet.

Introduction

Houseplants have been grown for centuries for their beauty, but something you may not know is that many houseplants, from aloe vera to orchids to popular ferns, also have powerful health benefits for you and your home.

In *Houseplants for a Healthy Home*, you'll find the profiles of fifty different houseplants—from the common aloe vera plant to the exotic chocolate oncidium orchid—that boast impressive health-giving qualities. Some of them purify indoor air of harmful toxins. Others are great for making tonics, poultices, and tinctures that can be used to treat all manner of conditions, from stomach upset to skin irritation to blocked sinuses. Each plant has been chosen specifically for its air-purifying power, unique physical features, or medicinal properties.

Each plant is presented in a colorfully illustrated profile that tells you everything you need to know about its health benefits. Profiles also include physical descriptions and size expectations—as well as in-depth information on water, temperature, and light needs—plus special growing tips. Best of all, you don't have to be an expert or buy specialized equipment to grow the plants in this book. In most cases, a sunny windowsill, a watering can, and a handful of fertilizer are all you need. And whether you're just starting to keep plants or have been growing them for years, you'll find a chapter full of everything you need to know to be successful, including common terms and definitions, information on what you should have on hand, and ten simple rules for successfully growing beautiful and healthy houseplants.

With all this information and more, *Houseplants for a Healthy Home* is guaranteed to help you gain a green thumb—and a beautiful, healthy home!

How to Care for Your Houseplants

Before your houseplants can take care of you and your home, you have to take care of them! Fortunately, keeping healthy houseplants isn't complicated. We've laid out the tools, ten simple rules, and common plant and garden terms for keeping your plants lush all year round.

WHAT TO HAVE ON HAND

Indoor gardening isn't complicated, but there are some important differences between growing plants inside and in an outdoor garden. Indoor plants can't just grow bigger roots to seek out more nutrients when they're hungry. Your house is also designed for you, not for your plants. This means air-conditioning, lower humidity, and a lack of proper sunlight. But not to worry: with the right tools, you can create a great indoor environment for your houseplants.

MATERIALS

As an indoor gardener you're lucky: you don't need a shed full of special equipment to keep your houseplants thriving. Instead, here are a few helpful tools to keep handy:

- **VARIOUS-SIZED CONTAINERS.** The most important thing with any indoor container is drainage. You can use clay, plastic, ceramic, or just about any other kind of pot, as long as it provides a way for water to drain out.
- **A WATERING CAN.** Any standard watering can found at your local hardware store will do.
- **GARDEN SHEARS.** Kitchen scissors will work for softer plants, but a good pair of sharp shears is ideal. Always keep shears clean.
- **SPRAY BOTTLES.** Consider getting a bottle for misting with pure water and a separate bottle for growth agents like neem oil or foliar feeding. Label your bottles so you don't mix them up.
- **GLOVES.** These are handy for keeping your hands clean when repotting plants.

FERTILIZERS

The difference between sort-of-healthy houseplants and lush, gorgeous houseplants is fertilizer. Since indoor plants are grown in containers, they rely on you to provide all of their nutrients, especially the "big three": nitrogen, phosphorus, and potassium (the "NPK" on a fertilizer label). There are many products out there that promise their combinations of special vitamins and enzymes are necessary for healthy plants. For the most part, however, a basic fertilizer combined with regular watering and repotting will allow your houseplants to thrive.

Here are a few types of potting soil and fertilizer for well-fed houseplants:

- FORTIFIED POTTING SOIL. Many leading potting soils have fertilizer included. For most common plants, this will be enough "food" to last for six months, or even a full growing season.

- CONTROLLED-RELEASE FERTILIZER PELLETS. A high-quality, controlled-release fertilizer will include the major NPK nutrients, plus a host of micronutrients, and will supply your plants with a continuous food supply for months. Follow the label directions to make sure you're using the right amount.

- LIQUID FERTILIZER. Many expert growers use liquid fertilizer because it's rapidly absorbed, easier to control in terms of dosing, and convenient. Look for one designed for houseplants and follow the label directions. If you really want to make your plants happy, use a little liquid fertilizer with every feeding during the growing season.

TEN TIPS FOR GROWING GREAT HOUSEPLANTS

The plants in this book can all be successfully grown indoors without taking any extraordinary measures. Still, if you're new to indoor gardening, it can take a little practice to get the hang of it. To help you out, we've provided a few simple guidelines that will apply to most plants. While each plant profile will have specific instructions for proper care, these are the basics:

1. USE A HIGH-QUALITY POTTING MEDIA. Never use gardening soil for indoor plants. Common "dirt" is far too heavy and provides poor drainage. A good potting media should include a lightweight base like

sphagnum peat moss or coconut coir to retain water, something to add structure like pine bark fines, and something that will increase drainage like perlite. Bagged potting soil might also contain added fertilizer and water-retention crystals, which will hold moisture longer so you don't have to water your plants as frequently.

2. BEWARE OF OLD DIRT. Bagged potting soils are not meant to last forever. Over time, the peat breaks down and becomes more acidic. The bigger chunks crumble into smaller, denser particles that compress around the plant's feeder roots, making the plant less able to take up water and oxygen. It won't be long before your container is filled with mostly roots, decomposed and exhausted potting media, and not much else. Repot plants annually for the best results.

3. LEARN TO WATER CORRECTLY. Improper watering is the number one killer of indoor plants. Overwatering can lead to decay and root rot, while underwatering can leave your plant dry and cause it to waste away. Never let your plants sit in water! After watering, let the container drain into its saucer, then empty the saucer of extra water.

4. LOOK FOR WAYS TO INCREASE HUMIDITY. Indoor environments are often heated or air-conditioned and have a very low humidity level, especially compared to the tropical regions where many of our favorite houseplants come from. Increase the humidity around your plants by filling a spray bottle with water and misting the leaves of your plant regularly.

5. USE FERTILIZER. Your container-bound plants rely on you to provide all of their nutrients, so invest in a good fertilizer, such as controlled-release pellets or liquid fertilizer.

6. KEEP AN EYE OUT FOR PESTS. The most common pests that affect indoor houseplants are aphids, mealybugs, whiteflies, scale insects, and spider mites. If you see pests, start with nonchemical solutions like isolating the affected plant and spraying it with water to blast the pests away. If you must use a pesticide, opt for the least toxic solution possible and always read the label to make sure the pesticide is approved for the type of insect you have and is safe for indoor use.

Neem oil is a popular choice for indoor plants. You can also use soapy water in a spray bottle, garlic and hot pepper sprays, or insecticides containing an ingredient called pyrethrum. In every case, it's always a good idea to first research the kind of bug you're fighting.

7. KEEP YOUR PLANTS CLEAN. Wiping the leaves clean with a moist cloth or paper towel will help keep your plants' pores open so they can absorb carbon dioxide more efficiently. This is especially important if you're using houseplants to help purify your air. For optimal air purification, you will need one plant for every 100 square feet of indoor space. Refer to the plant entries and appendix to discover the best air purifiers for your home.

8. USE THE RIGHT SIZE CONTAINER. Plants should be firmly rooted in their containers. If you see roots spilling over the edges of the container or growing from the drainage holes, it's time to repot. Likewise, if your plants are too heavy and tip over, you should consider repotting. When you repot, go up by one pot size at a time so the plant doesn't put too much energy into root growth at the expense of leaf growth.

9. MIMIC THE PLANT'S NATIVE ENVIRONMENT. If you're growing desert succulents, don't treat them like rainforest aroids, with high humidity and excessive watering. Instead, try to mimic the plant's natural desert habitat: bright light, sandy soil, low humidity, and low to moderate watering. A plant's native habitat will provide invaluable clues on how to grow it.

10. PAY ATTENTION! Don't worry too much about the "rules." Every house is slightly different, and your growing environment won't be the same as your neighbor's. Instead, get in the habit of paying attention to your plants. When you're watering or misting, peek at some leaf bottoms to see if any pests are snacking on your plants. Wiggle the stems to make sure your plants are well rooted. Are the leaf margins turning brown? Are leaves turning yellow and dropping off? Learn how to "read" the clues your plant is giving you so that you can cultivate healthy, happy healers.

HELPFUL TERMS TO KNOW

As you read through the plant profiles in this book, you may run into some words you haven't heard of before. Here you'll find a quick glossary of common plant and gardening terms that appear in this book. An asterisk beside a word indicates that you can refer to that word elsewhere in the glossary.

ANNUAL: A plant whose life cycle lasts one year before it produces new seeds and dies.

AROID: A plant from the Araceae family (also known as the arum family). The family is characterized by small flowers growing on a spike (spadix*) that is surrounded by a larger bract* (spathe*). Examples include the *Philodendron* and *Spathiphyllum* genera.

AYURVEDIC: A medical system that relies on herbal medications, special diets, and other homeopathic techniques to promote healing.

BRACT: A specialized type of leaf; a single flower emerges from the meeting point of the leaf and the plant stem.

BROMELIAD: A member of the family Bromeliaceae, usually an epiphyte* with a rosette* of fleshy leaves forming a central cup that holds water.

CANE: A hollow section or stalk of a plant (especially sugarcane, bamboo, and certain orchids).

CORM: An underground, enlarged stem used to store nutrients and water to help a plant survive adverse conditions, such as a dry season or winter.

DECOCTION: A concentrated extract made by boiling or heating plant parts, typically in water.

DORMANCY: The state when a plant temporarily stops growing. This typically occurs during the winter months.

EPIPHYTE: A type of plant that grows by attaching to a host plant, usually by its roots, but is not parasitic and does not usually harm the host plant. Examples include orchids and bromeliads*.

FROND: A leaf of a palm or fern, often containing multiple leaflets*.

HYBRID: A plant that is created when two related species or varieties are crossed together to form a third variety.

LEAFLET: A leaflike element or structure in a compound leaf. On a fern, the long fronds* are divided into many leaflets.

MARGIN: The edge of the leaf.

MIDRIB: The central vein of the leaf.

NODE: The section of a plant stem where a leaf or leaves emerge.

POULTICE: A preparation of plant material, usually leaves, that forms a moist, medicated bandage or covering and is applied directly to an affected area of the body.

PERENNIAL: A plant that grows each year through its natural life span.

PHYTOCHEMICAL: A substance derived from plants, often with medicinal properties.

POLYPHENOLS: Phytochemicals* that work as antioxidants in the body. Examples include quercetin and resveratrol, derived from red grapes.

PROPAGATE: To reproduce a plant, whether it's by seed or cuttings.

PSEUDOBULB: A bulb-like enlargement of a section of stem on an orchid, from which leaves and flowers emerge.

RHIZOME: A specialized type of underground stem that produces roots on the underside and sends up shoots from the upper side as it grows horizontally.

ROOT-BOUND: Occurs when a plant has outgrown its container so the roots have no more room to grow. Typically, the roots will form a tight ball that makes it difficult for the plant to absorb water, oxygen, and nutrients.

ROSETTE: A rose-shaped arrangement of leaves, particularly in bromeliads*.

SPADIX: A spike containing tiny flowers that occurs in the arum family (see *aroid**).

SPATHE: A large specialized leaf (bract*) that surrounds a spike of tiny flowers (spadix*) and occurs in the arum family (see *aroid**).

SUCCULENT: A plant with fleshy leaves or stems designed to store water to withstand drought or dry conditions. Examples include aloe vera and Chinese jade plants.

TINCTURE: A solution or extract prepared with an alcohol solvent.

TONIC: A medicine or substance that heals or invigorates you.

UNDERSTORY: The area of a forest under the main overhead tree canopy. Typically, the understory receives less direct sunlight and is warmer than the canopy.

The Plants

Aloe Vera

Aloe vera

DESCRIPTION

Upright with thick, gel-filled, pale green leaves lined with small teeth.

SIZE

Typically under 2' tall indoors.

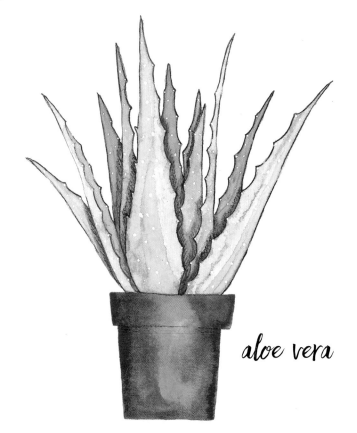

aloe vera

- Contains powerful antioxidants
- Promotes healthy skin
- Promotes healthy hair
- Fights inflammation
- Fights bacterial infections
- Fights heart disease and cancer
- Combats type 2 diabetes
- Fights gastric ulcers
- Promotes oral hygiene
- Promotes gastrointestinal health

Aloe vera has been harvested and cultivated for centuries, thanks to the long list of healing properties this spiky little plant offers. The gel is packed with over seventy-five powerful antioxidants, amino acids, and vitamins. An aloe vera tonic is used to reduce inflammation and bacterial infections; aid digestion; and help fight cancer, type 2 diabetes, gastric ulcers, gum disease, and heart disease. It's even a laxative. To make your own aloe vera tonic, peel the skin and rind from aloe vera leaves and mix the clear gel with a citrus juice.

The leaf gel is also a popular skin treatment for burns, small cuts, and even dandruff. If you've ever split open an aloe vera leaf and smeared the fresh gel on a sunburn, you already know how soothing and cooling aloe vera gel is.

HOW TO GROW THIS PLANT

LIGHT: Low light to direct sunlight is preferred.

WATER: Water when dry, then let drain. Good drainage is essential, and don't overwater.

TEMPERATURE: Average to warm temperatures are best. Avoid cold drafts.

TIPS: When harvesting aloe vera, cut leaves with a sharp knife. Repot every other year.

Areca Palm

Dypsis lutescens

DESCRIPTION

Feathery and arching fronds borne on clusters of smooth trunks. Mature palms eventually form clumps, although they are frequently grown as single-trunk plants indoors.

SIZE

Up to 20' tall outdoors. Indoor height will be restricted by the pot size.

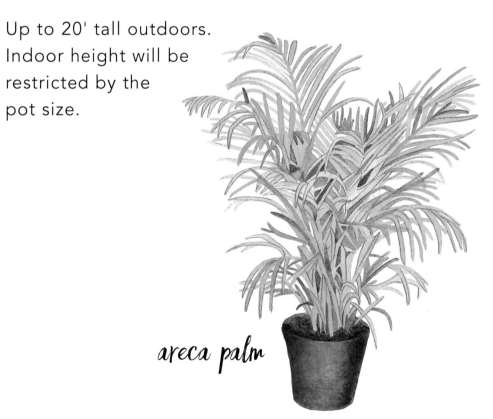

areca palm

∽ Removes airborne toxins   ∽ May promote weight loss

The areca palm isn't just a striking indoor palm; it's also one of the most powerful air-purifying plants, according to a NASA study published in 1989. Researchers singled out the areca palm for its ability to remove formaldehyde from the indoor environment. Formaldehyde is a skin irritant that has been linked to certain types of cancer and asthma. This common toxin is often "outgassed" from insulation and furniture products, meaning that it escapes from the material over time. Formaldehyde is also commonly found in cleaning products.

In addition to its air-purifying power, the areca palm may someday help fight obesity. One study showed that an extract of areca palm inhibited the "hunger hormone" in mice.

HOW TO GROW THIS PLANT

LIGHT: Provide bright, indirect sunlight. Avoid shady corners.

WATER: Regular, consistent watering and good drainage are essential.

TEMPERATURE: Warm and humid environments are ideal.

TIPS: Use a palm fertilizer according to label directions, and wipe leaves frequently to keep pores open for air purification.

Avocado

Persea americana

DESCRIPTION

Broad leaves up to 12" long, on a woody stem.

SIZE

Up to 20' outdoors. Indoors, size is determined by pot size and trimming.

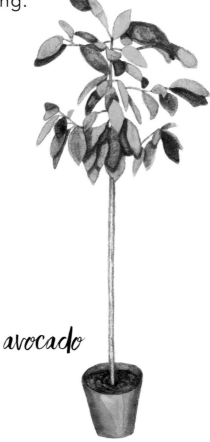

avocado

HEALTH BENEFITS

- Promotes healthy skin
- Eases aches and pains
- Lowers cholesterol
- May promote weight loss
- Promotes brain health
- Improves blood sugar levels

In Mexico and throughout the Caribbean, people have been brewing tea from avocado leaves for centuries, as well as making a poultice from the leaves. Modern researchers have found that avocado leaf extracts can lower cholesterol and fight obesity, reduce hunger, boost brain health, help maintain normal blood glucose levels, and reduce the inflammation that contributes to eczema and joint pain. To make avocado tea, boil a handful of avocado leaves in a cup or two of water for three minutes, then let steep. Strain out the leaves and add your favorite sweetener.

HOW TO GROW THIS PLANT

LIGHT: Direct sunlight is best.

WATER: Water weekly.

TEMPERATURE: A warm environment is best.

TIPS: Sprouting an avocado pit can be as simple as suspending the pit over a glass of water, making sure about 1" of the pit is in the water, and waiting for roots and leaves to emerge in about six weeks. Pot the young plant into dirt.

Bamboo Palm

Chamaedorea seifrizii

DESCRIPTION

Long stems with prominent nodes that resemble bamboo, topped with arching fronds that have long, drooping leaflets.

SIZE

Can grow to 7' outdoors but can be maintained at 4' indoors.

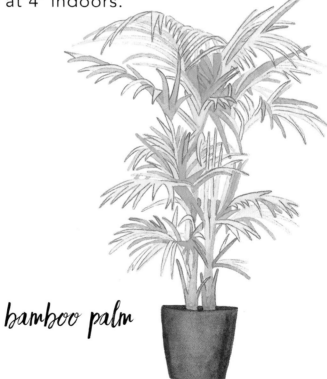

bamboo palm

🌿 Removes airborne toxins   🌿 Increases humidity

The graceful little bamboo palm is one of the most effective plants known for removing toxins such as trichloroethylene (TCE), benzene, and formaldehyde from the air. These are industrial toxins found in cleaning products and manufactured home furniture, and are linked to asthma, respiratory problems, and even an increased risk of cancer. In a controlled lab setting, the bamboo palm removed almost as much airborne formaldehyde as the study's most effective plant, the Janet Craig (*Dracaena deremensis* 'Janet Craig'). Combine bamboo palms with aroids and other palms to get extra air-purifying power. The bamboo palm also increases humidity, making it a great addition to your traditional humidifier.

HOW TO GROW THIS PLANT

☀ **LIGHT:** Dappled or low light is best.

💧 **WATER:** Keep continuously moist, but never let sit in water.

● **TEMPERATURE:** Warm, humid conditions are ideal. Cold drafts can cause leaf browning.

❋ **TIPS:** Provide a high-quality palm fertilizer according to label directions, and regularly flush the soil to remove built-up fertilizer salts. Repot mature plants every other year, or as needed.

Banana

Musa species

DESCRIPTION

Large, dramatic leaves unfurl from a central pseudostem in succession.

SIZE

Depends on the variety. Look for dwarf bananas for indoor growth, especially the Dwarf Cavendish. Mature plants will reach 5'.

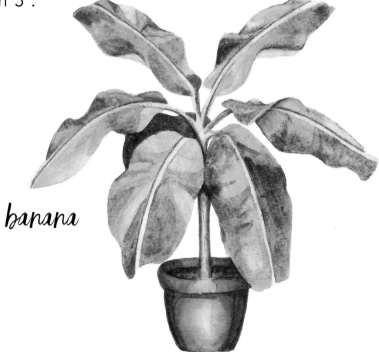

banana

- Reduces cold and flu symptoms
- Combats type 2 diabetes
- Treats respiratory conditions
- Promotes healthy skin
- Fights gastric ulcers

Banana leaves, roots, and flowers boast many health benefits, thanks to the dozens of healthy compounds in every part of the plant. In traditional Indian medicine, banana flowers are boiled in a tea and used to treat bronchitis, stomach ulcers, and type 2 diabetes. Banana leaves can be soaked in cold water and used as a poultice to relieve mild burns, while banana leaf tea provides relief for an inflamed throat. To make banana leaf tea, boil fresh leaves in water, then strain.

HOW TO GROW THIS PLANT

LIGHT: Provide bright light, including direct sunlight.

WATER: Water weekly.

TEMPERATURE: Warm, humid conditions are ideal.

TIPS: The rhizomes, or immature plants, are easily purchased online (growing bananas from seed is difficult), and growing your own bananas at home is incredibly rewarding. If your banana plant is healthy enough to send out shoots, let them grow until the first true leaves begin to emerge, then carefully cut the rhizome and repot.

Barberton Daisy

Gerbera jamesonii

DESCRIPTION

Diamond-shaped, thin-textured leaves with slightly serrated edges. Flowers are borne on stalks and are available in many bold colors.

SIZE

Low-growing (less than 12" tall) with flowers that can rise another 12".

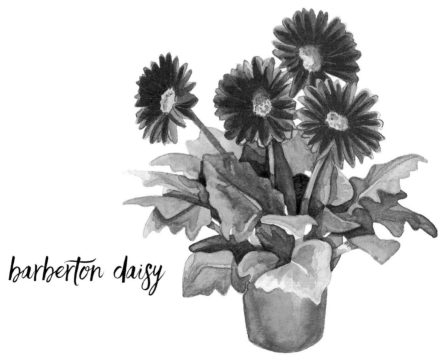

barberton daisy

HEALTH BENEFITS

❧ Removes airborne toxins   ❧ Increases nighttime oxygen

The Barberton daisy, also known as the gerbera daisy, was included in a NASA clean air study, published in 1989, as one of the most effective air purifiers. The scientists found that Barberton daisies were effective in removing trichloroethylene (TCE) and benzene from the environment. These toxins are found in manufactured home goods and many cleaning agents, and cause health issues such as difficulty breathing, headaches, and nausea.

Unlike most plants, the Barberton daisy releases oxygen at night. Move the plant to your nightstand before bed for more breathable air.

HOW TO GROW THIS PLANT

LIGHT: A sunny windowsill is perfect. Avoid low-light, north-facing exposures.

WATER: Keep soil regularly moist. Look for signs of wilt, and water immediately. You can extend flowering by using a diluted liquid fertilizer every week. Refer to the fertilizer label for instructions.

TEMPERATURE: Moderate temperatures up to 75°F are ideal. Beware of direct, cold drafts, which will cause flowers to die more quickly.

TIPS: Remove old flowers to keep the plant healthy and flourishing. When the flowers are spent, grow as a regular houseplant until next year's flowering season.

Basil

Ocimum basilicum

DESCRIPTION

Smooth, dark green leaves. Flowers are small and white and borne on upright stalks.

SIZE

Reaches a maximum height of 18" before flowering.

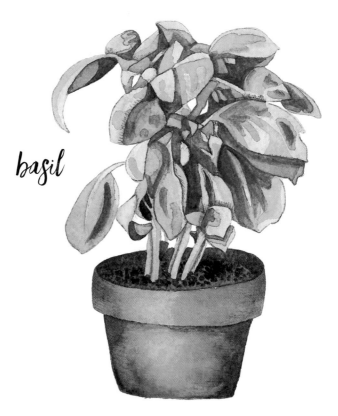

basil

- Fights inflammation
- Fights depression
- Reduces stress
- Promotes gastrointestinal health

- Antimicrobial
- Antibacterial
- Contains powerful antioxidants

Native to tropical Asia, basil is found in cuisines across the world and used in holistic medicines, including Ayurvedic medicine. The plant provides a wide range of vitamins and minerals that combat stress and depression. Basil oil has also been shown to kill bacteria and microbes.

Basil leaves are rich in polyphenols (chemicals that fight cell-damaging molecules) and essential oils that fight inflammation, including arthritis. Basil leaves can also be used to make an herbal tea that helps to relieve stomach upset. To make basil tea, steep fresh or dried leaves in boiling water for three minutes, then strain and drink.

HOW TO GROW THIS PLANT

LIGHT: Provide four hours of direct sunlight per day.

WATER: Regular watering is needed. Water wilted plants immediately.

TEMPERATURE: Temperate or warm rooms are preferred.

TIPS: Potted basil is commonly sold in the produce section of supermarkets and grocery stores, but the plant is also easily started from seed. Older basil or basil that has started flowering loses its pungency and flavor, so it's best to use basil when it's still young. Pinch off growing tips with a pair of sharp scissors or shears to prolong the plant's useful life.

Boston Fern

Nephrolepis exaltata 'Bostoniensis'

DESCRIPTION

Long, arching, and somewhat brittle fronds with small alternate leaflets along the midrib.

SIZE

Fronds will grow up to 3' long.

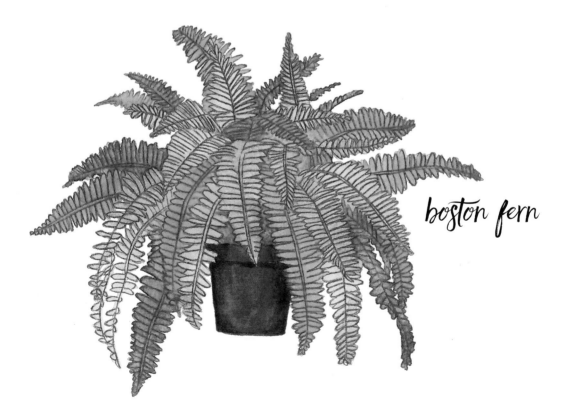

boston fern

🌿 Removes airborne toxins   🌿 Increases humidity

Among the oldest plants on the planet, ferns are prized for their ability to remove airborne pollutants, especially formaldehyde, xylene, and toluene. These common industrial toxins are found in household cleaners and manufactured furniture, and can lead to health issues such as headaches, trouble breathing, and the growth of cancerous cells. The Boston fern is also good at raising indoor humidity, which can help soothe dry and wintry nasal passages.

HOW TO GROW THIS PLANT

LIGHT: Indirect sunlight is ideal. Some morning or early evening direct sunlight is okay.

WATER: Water weekly and mist daily.

TEMPERATURE: Ideal temperatures are between 65°F and 75°F.

TIPS: Boston ferns are among the most common indoor ferns, partly because they aren't as tricky to take care of as some other fern species. They grow particularly well as hanging plants or when placed on decorative columns. During the summer growing season, they respond well to weekly applications of a liquid fertilizer. The plants don't mind being pot-bound, so you should repot only once every other year. Divide the plant during repotting.

Bromeliads

Various genera, including *Aechmea*, *Vriesea*, and *Guzmania*

DESCRIPTION

Low rosettes of strappy leaves surrounding a central "cup" that contains water. The leaves may have sharp serrations and should be handled with care. Impressive flowering bracts rise above the plant.

SIZE

Reaches a maximum height of 18" indoors, with 2' flower bracts.

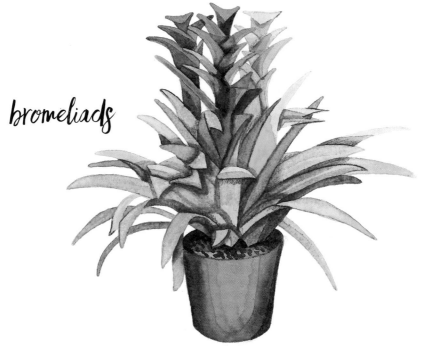

bromeliads

✎ Removes airborne toxins   ✎ Increases daytime oxygen

These spiky little epiphytes are not edible (with one famous exception—the pineapple!) or particularly striking; however, in a study conducted at the State University of New York at Oswego, bromeliads were found to be extremely effective at removing volatile organic compounds (VOCs) from the air. Scientists singled out acetone, the toxin used in nail polish remover, and found that bromeliads removed 80 percent of acetone from the air. Bromeliads also purify indoor air of formaldehyde, benzene, toluene, xylene, and styrene. These harmful VOCs can be found in manufactured furniture and household cleaners, and increase the risk of cancer and asthma symptoms. Keeping a few bromeliads is also a great way to increase the oxygen levels in your home.

HOW TO GROW THIS PLANT

LIGHT: Indirect sunlight is ideal.

WATER: Water by filling up the central cup with clean water as needed.

TEMPERATURE: Warm rooms are ideal. Avoid cold drafts and temperatures below 50°F.

TIPS: Bromeliad bracts may last several months indoors. When the bract begins to die, trim it by cutting close to the base. The mother plant will slowly die after the bract dies, but if you continue to water and care for the plant, it may put out small plantlets that can be repotted.

Chinese Evergreen

Aglaonema modestum

DESCRIPTION

Evergreen perennial featuring a crown of oval leaves, sometimes with striking variegation in light green and silver.

SIZE

Slow-growing, reaching up to 2' tall indoors.

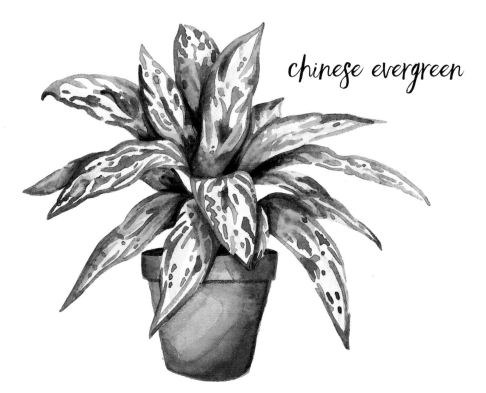

chinese evergreen

🌿 Removes airborne toxins   🌿 Increases daytime oxygen

The Chinese evergreen has more going for it than just its beautiful foliage and its reputation as a good luck plant in China. In research studies, the Chinese evergreen was shown to increase oxygen while removing the industrial toxins formaldehyde and benzene from indoor air. Formaldehyde has been linked to respiratory problems and an increased risk of cancer, and is found in household cleaners and furniture. Benzene is present in a wide variety of common household objects, including ink, oil, paint, plastics, and rubber. It's also used in the manufacturing process to create detergents, dyes, and some pharmaceuticals. This common chemical can cause irritation of sensitive tissues in the eyes and skin, and it's a known carcinogen according to the American Cancer Society.

Be aware that no part of this plant should ever be consumed, either by people or animals, as it's mildly toxic and can cause irritation and swelling.

HOW TO GROW THIS PLANT

✳️ **LIGHT:** Low light is preferred. Avoid exposure to direct sunlight.

💧 **WATER:** Water weekly during the summer growing season. In winter, water when the top 1" of soil is dry.

⬤ **TEMPERATURE:** Ideal temperatures are above 70°F. Leaf damage may begin in mid-60s (°F).

❋ **TIPS:** During the growing season, use a controlled-release fertilizer for best results. Follow the fertilizer label instructions.

Chinese Jade Plant

Crassula ovata

DESCRIPTION

Perennial shrub with dark green, fleshy leaves on branched stems. Scented flowers occur in pink or white clusters.

SIZE

Slow-growing, reaching up to 3' tall.

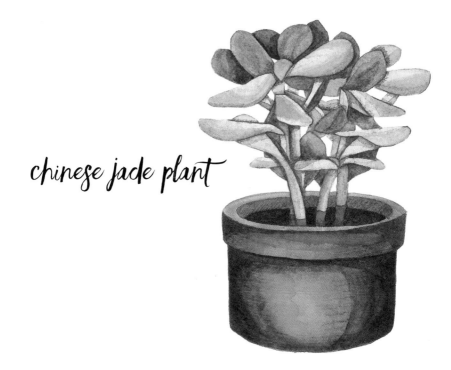

chinese jade plant

HEALTH BENEFITS

- Promotes healthy skin
- Promotes gastrointestinal health

In China, the jade plant is considered a powerful symbol of good luck and is used extensively in feng shui, the ancient practice of arranging objects to create a positive energy flow. These African succulents also boast some interesting health benefits. In African folk medicine, the leaves are used to cure common warts. To treat a wart, a leaf is split open to expose the gel-like interior, then wrapped over the wart and left for three days. If the treatment is successful, the wart will fall off. The Khoi tribe in Africa also boils the leaves in milk as a remedy for diarrhea and stomach queasiness. This plant may be toxic for animals, however, so keep it away from your pets.

HOW TO GROW THIS PLANT

LIGHT: Dappled light is preferred. Plants exposed to more sunlight may have a reddish tint or even a slightly yellow cast.

WATER: Water sparingly and never let sit in water. When watering, drench the soil and then let dry completely. Good drainage is essential.

TEMPERATURE: Moderate temperatures—mid-70s (°F)—are preferred, but it can adjust in near freezing temperatures.

TIPS: Jade plants are very resilient houseplants that can live for decades. Dust their leaves occasionally to keep them glossy, and beware of brittle branches that can break easily under pressure.

Chocolate Oncidium

Oncidium 'Sharry Baby'

DESCRIPTION

Large, oblong, upright pseudobulbs that rise from a mass of thin, white roots. Narrow, strappy leaves emerge from the top of the pseudobulb. Flower spikes appear in the fall.

SIZE

Leaves can be up to 2' long, with 3' flower spikes that are covered with small, intricate flowers that smell exactly like chocolate.

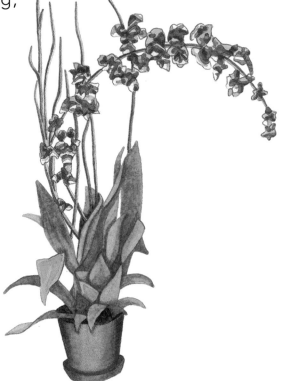

chocolate oncidium

HEALTH BENEFITS

✎ Removes airborne toxins   ✎ Increases daytime oxygen

While refreshing the air with its delicious scent, the chocolate oncidium is also purifying it. Oncidiums have been shown to remove toxins such as formaldehyde from indoor air. Formaldehyde is found in manufactured goods, such as furniture, industrial resins, and home cleaning agents, and can cause headaches and respiratory problems. This orchid further purifies indoor air by releasing oxygen into your home during daylight hours.

HOW TO GROW THIS PLANT

LIGHT: Moderate to bright light is ideal. Oncidiums are more forgiving of direct sunlight than many other orchids.

WATER: Water daily during the summer growing season and reduce watering in winter to once a week. Immaculate drainage is essential, and the plant should completely dry out between waterings. The more exposed the roots are, the more frequently you need to water, but never let the orchid sit in standing water.

TEMPERATURE: Intermediate to warm temperatures are best. Plants will go dormant below 50°F.

TIPS: These plants can be successfully grown in slatted pots or even tied to a mount.

Christmas Cactus

Schlumbergera bridgesii

DESCRIPTION

Drooping "branches" made from flattened segments of stem. Flowers emerge from stem tips. Available in multiple colors, but red is traditional.

SIZE

Branches can reach 3' in length.

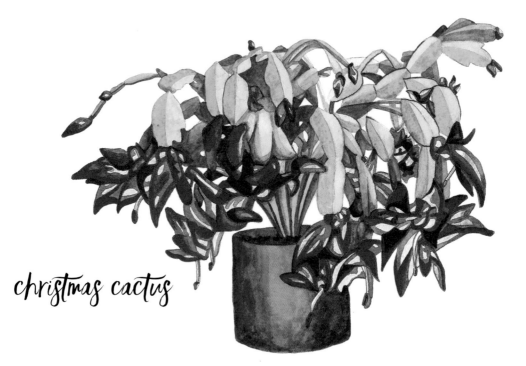

christmas cactus

✎ Removes airborne toxins   ✎ Increases nighttime oxygen

This showy, tropical cactus is an effective air-purifying plant that filters out indoor toxins, including formaldehyde, benzene, and toluene. These toxins are found in many manufactured home goods, such as furniture and cleaning supplies, and can cause issues such as nausea and shortness of breath.

Unlike many plants, the Christmas cactus releases oxygen at night instead of throughout the day. Position the plant in your bedroom to increase oxygen levels while you sleep.

HOW TO GROW THIS PLANT

LIGHT: Dappled light is ideal. During the winter months, aim for some direct sunlight.

WATER: Mist daily and keep soil evenly moist. Never let sit in water.

TEMPERATURE: Average room temperature is preferred.

TIPS: Christmas cacti blooms are triggered by the amount of light versus darkness (the photoperiod). After the winter bloom is done and the flowers have fallen off, cut back on watering and fertilizer—water only when the top 1" of soil is dry or if the plant shows signs of water distress (e.g. wrinkled leaves). As soon as it starts to grow again, keep the plant at 50°F–55°F and provide fourteen hours of total darkness. Buds will soon appear, and you can then move the plant back to a warmer room and resume regular watering.

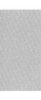

Crocus

Crocus sativus

DESCRIPTION

Long green leaves sprout in midsummer, followed by striking purple flowers in the fall and a period of vegetative growth characterized by longer, strappy leaves.

SIZE

Reaches up to 1' tall.

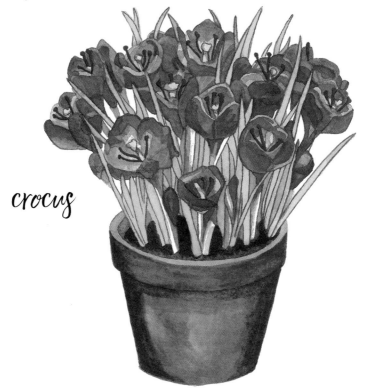

crocus

HEALTH BENEFITS

- Treats respiratory conditions
- Promotes sleep
- Fights heart disease and cancer
- Contains powerful antioxidants
- Reduces PMS symptoms

The beautiful, fall-blooming *Crocus sativus* is the source of saffron, a spice that is made by harvesting the red stigma, or "thread" that appears in the center of the flower, and gently drying it. Saffron is loaded with antioxidants and dozens of healthy phytochemicals that treat respiratory conditions such as asthma and bronchitis, insomnia, cancer, heart disease, and premenstrual syndrome symptoms.

When buying this plant, be careful that you're not confusing it with the autumn crocus (*Colchicum autumnale*), which is toxic.

HOW TO GROW THIS PLANT

LIGHT: Moderate to bright light is needed during the flowering and vegetative season, which begins in the fall and lasts through the spring.

WATER: Water weekly during winter once small, grasslike leaves have emerged. Water every other day during spring vegetative growth.

TEMPERATURE: Corms require a period of cold (around 40°F) during the fall and winter months to begin vegetative growth. During the spring vegetative period, keep the plant in a cool room. The leaves will shrivel up and disappear, then new flowers will emerge from the corm in late summer, beginning the cycle once again.

TIPS: Start crocus corms in shallow pots filled with a loose potting mixture.

Dendrobium

Dendrobium nobile

DESCRIPTION

Pseudobulbs produce upright, stiff canes with short, stiff leaves. Flower spikes emerge from canes and bear white or purple flowers.

SIZE

Canes reach up to 2' in height, with flower spikes as long as 2'.

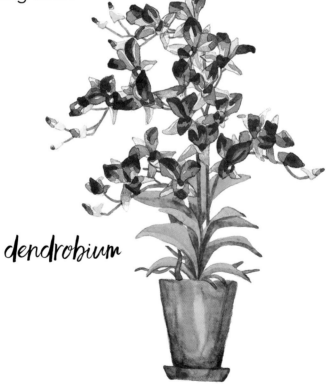

dendrobium

- May promote weight loss
- Promotes gastrointestinal health
- Promotes brain health
- Boosts immune system
- Improves blood sugar levels

A mainstay in traditional Chinese medicine, the leaves and dried stems of dendrobium orchids can be used to brew teas that boost the immune system, promote weight loss, protect the brain from proteins linked to Alzheimer's disease, regulate blood sugar, and reduce stomach upset. To make the tea, boil the stems and leaves in water for ten minutes, then let sit for another five minutes before drinking.

HOW TO GROW THIS PLANT

LIGHT: Filtered light is best. Avoid direct sunlight.

WATER: Water once daily or every other day during the summer growing season. The winter watering schedule will depend on your growing method. If you're growing on a plaque or mount, water once a week or less. If you're growing in a pot, water every other week. Good drainage is essential.

TEMPERATURE: Cool temperatures (between 55°F and 65°F) in the fall or winter will stimulate a flower spike. During the growing season, keep moderately warm.

TIPS: Once flowers have faded, cut off the spike near the base. Old canes will eventually die, but new canes will emerge at the base of the pseudobulb. Repot when the plant overgrows the sides of its container.

Dracaena deremensis 'Janet Craig'

Dracaena deremensis 'Janet Craig'

DESCRIPTION

Long, tapered, solid green leaves borne on multiple stems. Leaves have slight ridges.

SIZE

Slow-growing, reaching up to 8' tall.

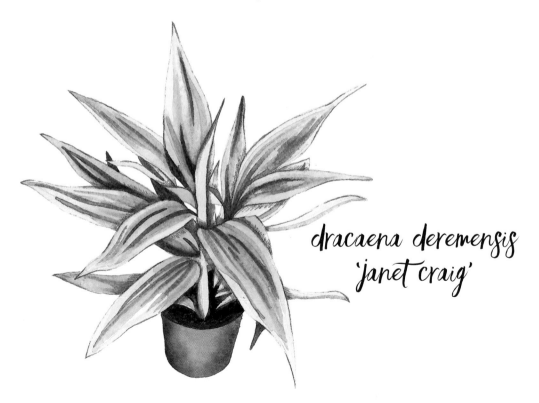

dracaena deremensis
'janet craig'

Removes airborne toxins   Increases daytime oxygen

Known as the Janet Craig, this member of the *Dracaena* genus is a work-horse when it comes to purifying the air in your environment and increasing oxygen levels. According to a major study by NASA, the Janet Craig was the most effective plant at removing trichloroethylene (TCE), benzene, and formaldehyde toxins from the air. These industrial toxins are found in manufactured home products and can cause headaches, respiratory conditions, and an increased risk of cancer. If you have room for only one type of plant to purify your air, this is the one to buy. Like other *Dracaena* species, this plant may be mildly toxic for animals, so keep it away from pets.

HOW TO GROW THIS PLANT

LIGHT: Moderate to low light is ideal. Leaf narrowing over time is a sign of inadequate light.

WATER: Water weekly, but don't soak. This plant can tolerate mild drought. Many experts advise using nonfluoridated water. Mist the leaves once daily or every few days to provide extra humidity. If conditions get too arid, the leaf tips may turn brown.

TEMPERATURE: Average room temperature is ideal. Avoid cold drafts.

TIPS: Use a controlled-release fertilizer at the beginning of the summer growing season. Follow fertilizer label instructions.

Dracaena deremensis 'Warneckii'

Dracaena deremensis 'Warneckii'

DESCRIPTION

Stiff, arching leaves emerge from upright, cane-like stems. Plants are often multistemmed. Leaves feature a central stripe, usually in gray or white.

SIZE

Can reach 8' in height, with leaves growing up to 12" long.

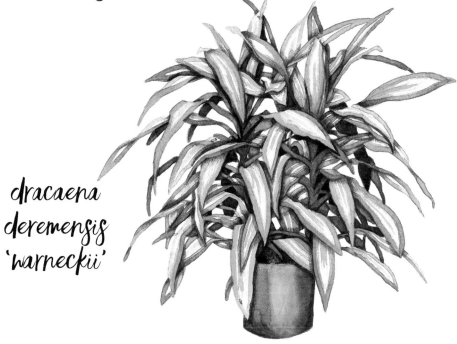

dracaena deremensis 'warneckii'

🌿 Removes airborne toxins   🌿 Increases daytime oxygen

The *D. deremensis* 'Warneckii' is a living air filter. This houseplant was studied by NASA and was found to remove up to 50 percent of benzene and formaldehyde from the indoor environment. These household toxins are used in the manufacture of everyday products and are "outgassed" (released into the air) by furniture and other items. *D. deremensis* 'Warneckii' has also been found to remove 10 percent of airborne trichloroethylene (TCE), a harmful chemical compound used in industrial solvents. TCE can cause respiratory issues, as well as headaches and nausea.

This purifier also releases oxygen during daylight hours to increase oxygen levels. The *D. deremensis* 'Warneckii' may be mildly toxic for animals, however, so don't allow your pets to eat its leaves.

HOW TO GROW THIS PLANT

LIGHT: Low to moderate light is ideal.

WATER: Weekly watering is best, but moderate drought is tolerated. Keep well drained.

TEMPERATURE: Average room temperature is best.

TIPS: These are tough plants that can thrive on benign neglect. Use a controlled-release fertilizer twice a year or weekly liquid fertilizer to achieve best results. Repot the plant annually to refresh the soil, and root-prune larger plants so they don't outgrow their containers.

Dracaena fragrans 'Massangeana'

Dracaena fragrans 'Massangeana'

DESCRIPTION

Single canes or groups of canes with leaves emerging from the top or branches. Leaves are wide and drooping, with lighter stripes along the midrib.

SIZE

Canes can reach 6' or more, with arching leaves that grow up to 18" in length.

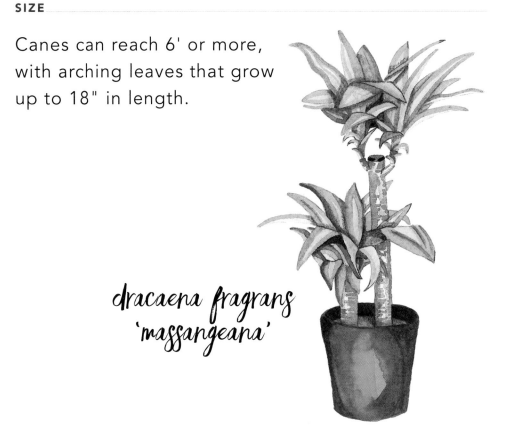

dracaena fragrans 'massangeana'

HEALTH BENEFITS

✿ Removes airborne toxins ✿ Increases daytime oxygen

Often called the corn plant or cornstalk plant, the *D. fragrans* 'Massangeana' is an excellent air purifier. This plant was shown to remove 70 percent of formaldehyde from the indoor environment in a clean air study by NASA, published in 1989. A common ingredient in household cleaners, formaldehyde contributes to a condition known as the "sick building syndrome." As buildings have become better insulated, formaldehyde and other toxins are trapped inside. When these toxins build up, symptoms like itching, coughing, nausea, dizziness, and headaches can occur.

The *D. fragrans* 'Massangeana' also increases oxygen levels in your home. Like other *Dracaena* species, however, this plant may be mildly toxic to animals, so keep it away from pets.

HOW TO GROW THIS PLANT

✼ **LIGHT:** Low to moderate light is ideal. Avoid too much direct sunlight, as strong light can wash out the leaf color.

💧 **WATER:** Water weekly and keep soil moist but well drained. It is also sensitive to fluoride in tap water, so it's best to use distilled or nonfluoridated water.

● **TEMPERATURE:** Moderate temperatures are perfect.

✳ **TIPS:** Check occasionally to make sure the canes are firmly rooted in the soil. Plants with loose canes should be repotted.

Dracaena marginata

Dracaena marginata

DESCRIPTION

Stiff, narrow, rapier-like leaves that grow from upright stems. The leaves are dark green with red margins, giving the plant an overall reddish cast. The Tricolor variety also features an ivory stripe.

SIZE

Multibranching stems can reach 10' in height. Indoor height depends on the container size. Leaves are up to 18" in length on mature plants.

dracaena marginata

Removes airborne toxins   Increases daytime oxygen

The *D. marginata* is a superior air-purifying plant, with the ability to remove benzene, trichloroethylene (TCE), and formaldehyde from indoor air. These harmful toxins have been linked to respiratory problems and an increased risk of cancer. To get the most air-purifying power from your plants, cluster multiple specimens together. The *D. marginata* also boosts oxygen levels in your home. Like other *Dracaena* species, however, the *D. marginata* may be mildly toxic to animals, so don't allow your pets to eat its leaves.

HOW TO GROW THIS PLANT

LIGHT: Low to moderate light is perfect. Too much sunlight will reduce color contrast on the leaves.

WATER: Relatively drought tolerant. Keep soil moist but not wet. This plant is sensitive to fluoride and salt, so it's recommended to use distilled or nonfluoridated water and regularly flush the soil to remove accumulated fertilizer salts.

TEMPERATURE: A warm room is ideal.

TIPS: The *D. marginata* has a slightly higher need for fertilization than other members of *Dracaena*, so biannual applications of a quality controlled-release fertilizer or weekly applications of a liquid fertilizer are a good idea.

Dumb Cane

Dieffenbachia species

DESCRIPTION

Herbaceous perennials that feature alternate, oblong, and typically variegated leaves emerging from upright stems.

SIZE

Can reach 5' in height but commonly grow to between 2' and 3' indoors.

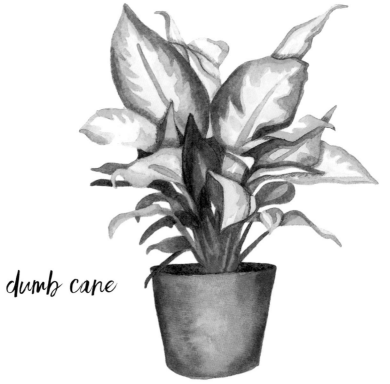

dumb cane

HEALTH BENEFITS

✎ Removes airborne toxins   ✎ Increases daytime oxygen

The *Dieffenbachia* plant, commonly known as the dumb cane, features large leaves that are more than just pretty. In a controlled laboratory experiment, a dumb cane plant was shown to be effective at removing ammonia and xylene from the indoor environment. In one study, dumb cane was shown to remove 325 micrograms of xylene per hour. Ammonia and xylene, which are used in household cleaners as well as manufacturing processes, have both been associated with respiratory issues, skin irritation, worsened asthma, and other ill health effects.

Dumb cane is also excellent for increasing oxygen levels in your home. Be careful when handling it, however, as contact with its milky sap can cause skin irritation, and the plant should never be consumed.

HOW TO GROW THIS PLANT

☀ **LIGHT:** Dappled shade or indirect sunlight is perfect. Avoid direct sunlight during the summer, as this may cause the leaves to brown.

💧 **WATER:** Keep soil continuously moist. In the winter, only water when the top 1" of soil is dry. Leaf browning may be a sign of improper watering.

⬤ **TEMPERATURE:** A warm, humid room is best. Low humidity can cause browning leaves.

✳ **TIPS:** During the winter, growth may slow, and it's common for the lower leaves to fall off over time.

Dwarf Date Palm

Phoenix roebelenii

DESCRIPTION

Drooping fronds covered with long, narrow leaflets top a slender trunk.

SIZE

Can grow up to 4' tall indoors, with fronds reaching
up to 3' in length.

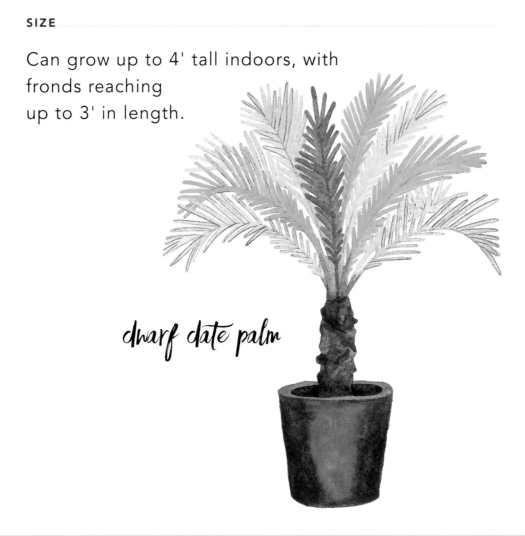

dwarf date palm

🌿 Removes airborne toxins   🌿 Increases daytime oxygen

The dwarf date palm is beautifully exotic—and it's great for your health. According to a study published by Dr. Bill Wolverton in the *Journal of the Mississippi Academy of Sciences*, this little palm filters out industrial toxins such as formaldehyde, xylene, and ammonia, which have been linked to respiratory issues and an increased risk of cancer. These chemicals are released in the home through manufactured furniture and cleaning products.

The dwarf date palm also increases oxygen levels in your home. Group plants together to boost their air-purifying power.

HOW TO GROW THIS PLANT

☀ **LIGHT:** Direct sunlight is ideal. Avoid low light.

💧 **WATER:** Semi-drought tolerant, but provide regular water during the summer growing season. Never let the palm sit in water, which can cause root rot. Mist leaves once daily or every few days to maintain humidity.

⬤ **TEMPERATURE:** Normal room temperature is best. Avoid cold drafts.

✳ **TIPS:** Fertilize once annually with a high-quality palm fertilizer. Dwarf date palms do better when they're slightly root-bound, so repot every other year or as necessary. Be careful not to disturb or damage roots during repotting. If the leaves start to turn yellow, supplement with magnesium sulfate (Epsom salt), mixed to a ratio of about ½ tablespoon per half gallon of water.

Dwarf French Lavender

Lavandula dentata

DESCRIPTION

Pale flowers borne on tall spikes and protected by distinctive purple bracts. Leaves are slightly fuzzy and deeply scalloped.

SIZE

Can grow up to 2' tall but reaches an average of 1' indoors.

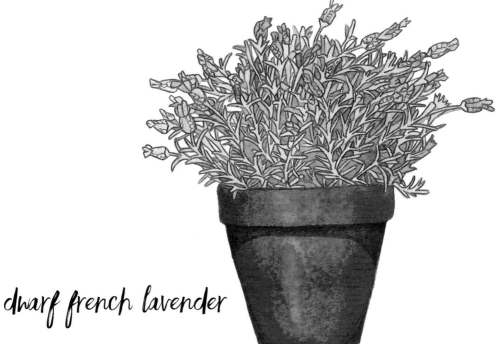

dwarf french lavender

HEALTH BENEFITS

- Reduces stress
- Aromatherapeutic
- Promotes sleep

Lavender has been cultivated for centuries for its simple beauty and wide range of health benefits. Modern research shows that the smell of lavender reduces stress and promotes calm, but if you've ever taken a deep breath of lavender in full bloom, you didn't need a scientist to tell you that!

Lavender leaves and flowers can be dried and used to make potpourris or sachets. You can also simmer lavender leaves and flowers to make lavender floral water, which can be put in a spray bottle and used as a room mist. Finally, the leaves and flowers are rich in plant polyphenols and can be used to make a soothing lavender tea before bed to help you sleep better.

HOW TO GROW THIS PLANT

LIGHT: Plenty of direct sunlight is necessary. Avoid north-facing windows.

WATER: Keep very well drained and never let water sit in the saucer.

TEMPERATURE: Average room temperature is ideal. Avoid temperatures below 50°F.

TIPS: Native to the Mediterranean, lavender thrives in a slightly alkaline, rocky soil. Add a pinch of lime to your potting mix to raise the pH. When the bloom is done, or the plant's stems have stretched out and are visible, you can transplant it outside.

Elephant Ear Philodendron

Philodendron domesticum

DESCRIPTION

A slow climber with spade-shaped, glossy, green leaves. Variegated types feature light green splashes on leaves.

SIZE

Leaves can be 12"–24" long but are around 6" in normal indoor conditions.

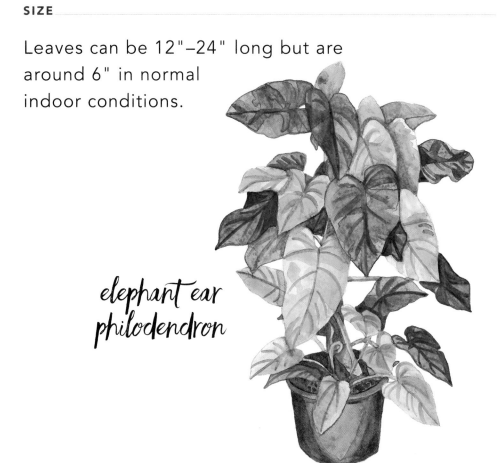

elephant ear philodendron

🍃 Removes hydrocarbons   🍃 Removes airborne toxins

Sometimes called the spade leaf philodendron, the elephant ear philodendron was praised by the University of Colorado for its ability to remove airborne toxins—especially formaldehyde, an ingredient in industrial cleaners that has been linked to respiratory ailments and an increased risk of cancer.

A study in the *International Journal of Engineering, Technology, Science and Research* also singled out the elephant ear philodendron for its ability to remove hydrocarbons, or emissions caused by burning oil and gasoline. These dangerous pollutants are known to increase the risk of cancer. Group elephant ear philodendrons with other aroids and palms to create a beautiful tropical display. Don't let children or pets snack on this plant, however, as all parts of the elephant ear philodendron are mildly toxic and can cause stomach upset.

HOW TO GROW THIS PLANT

LIGHT: Bright, filtered sunlight is ideal.

WATER: Keep continuously moist and mist the leaves daily. Wipe the leaves regularly to keep pores open for the most air-purifying power.

TEMPERATURE: Year-round warmth is ideal. Growth will slow in cold weather.

TIPS: There are many species of plants that go by the name "elephant ear." Make sure you look for the correct species name (*Philodendron domesticum*) so you know you're getting the plant with the greatest health benefits. Only repot when the plant is root-bound.

Emerald Gem

Homalomena rubra

DESCRIPTION

Dark and glossy green, heart-shaped leaves on a compact, low-growing stem.

SIZE

Leaves can reach up to 18" in perfect conditions.

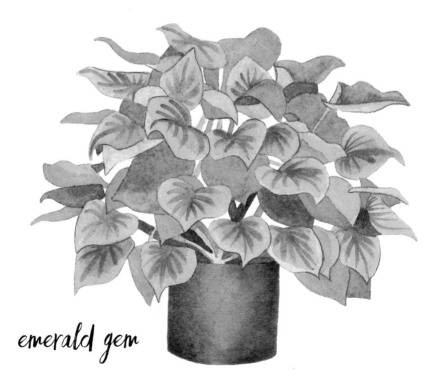

emerald gem

HEALTH BENEFITS

🌿 Removes airborne toxins   🌿 Increases daytime oxygen

The plant known as *Homalomena* 'Emerald Gem' was introduced in the 1980s. In air purification studies, species of *Homalomena* have been singled out for their ability to filter toxins from the air, including the industrial toxins ammonia, formaldehyde, and xylene, which have been linked to respiratory issues and even an increased risk of cancer. In a study published by the Mississippi Academy of Sciences, *Homalomena* species were especially effective at getting rid of ammonia. They are also used to increase oxygen levels indoors.

Other members of the *Homalomena* genus have been used in traditional Chinese and Tamil medicine for centuries, but never ingest any part of the common Emerald Gem.

HOW TO GROW THIS PLANT

☀ **LIGHT:** Bright, filtered sunlight is ideal.

💧 **WATER:** Water weekly.

⚫ **TEMPERATURE:** Keep in a warm room, with temperatures above 70°F.

✳ **TIPS:** The Emerald Gem grows well in a slightly undersized pot, and it's more sensitive to cold than many sources would have you believe. Distressed plants drop their leaves or experience leaf yellowing. Put the plant in a warm, bright, and humid place and give it some time to acclimate. Some leaves may drop while it's adjusting, but hang in there and don't move it! Once the plant is adjusted, it will be fine.

English Ivy

Hedera helix

DESCRIPTION

Perennial vines with dark green leaves that often feature white veins.

SIZE

Indoor height is limited to support size and pruning.

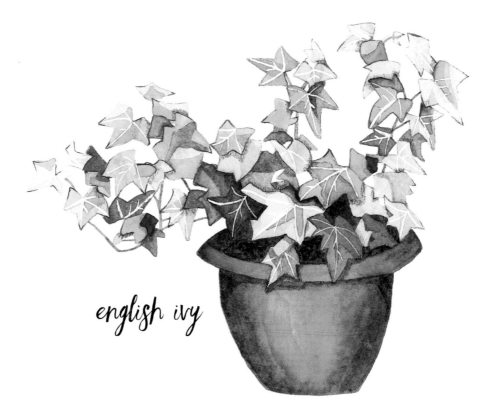

english ivy

HEALTH BENEFITS

- Removes airborne toxins
- Increases daytime oxygen
- Treats respiratory conditions
- Fights inflammation

English ivy is famous for its furious growth rate, which makes it excellent at producing oxygen and purifying the air of trichloroethylene (TCE), xylene, benzene, and formaldehyde. These harmful toxins are found in household cleaners and manufactured furniture, and can cause headaches, respiratory problems, and an increased risk of cancer.

English ivy extract has been used for centuries to treat respiratory conditions like asthma and bronchitis, as well as inflammation and allergic reactions. To make an extract, crush a handful of leaves with a mortar and pestle. Add ethyl alcohol and refrigerate overnight. Filter the mixture through a paper coffee filter multiple times, then store in the refrigerator. To use, mix the extract with water or take the drops directly. You can also steep the leaves in boiling water for ten minutes to make a tea. Don't consume large amounts of leaves directly, however, as the plant contains saponin, a chemical that can cause stomach upset and vomiting.

HOW TO GROW THIS PLANT

LIGHT: Bright, indirect sunlight is ideal, but it is tolerant of a wide range of light conditions.

WATER: Water weekly throughout the year.

TEMPERATURE: Average room temperatures are best, but it can tolerate colder temperatures.

TIPS: Provide a growing support for larger plants. Smaller specimens can be displayed as a trailing plant.

Eucalyptus

Eucalyptus globulus

DESCRIPTION

A large tree featuring drooping, fragrant leaves.

SIZE

Mature trees are over 60' tall. Indoor height is limited by container size and pruning.

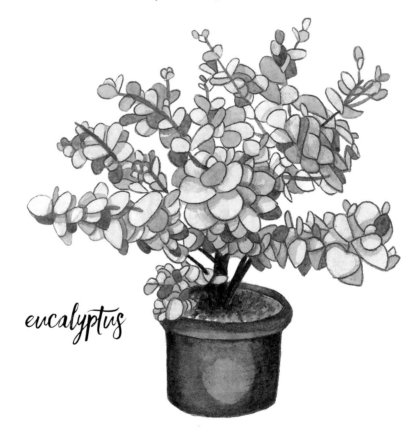

eucalyptus

HEALTH BENEFITS

- Treats respiratory conditions
- Promotes healthy skin
- Boosts immune system
- Antibacterial
- Reduces cold and flu symptoms

The eucalyptus tree contains dozens of powerful health-promoting compounds. Use eucalyptus essential oil on wounds to reduce the risk of bacterial infection, or massage into the chest to treat asthma. The oil can also be used to soothe burns and other skin irritations. To make eucalyptus oil, poach the leaves in olive oil over a low temperature for six hours (a slow-cooker is perfect), then strain the mixture until the leaves are separated from the oil. Mix the oil with warm water and use as a gargle to treat sore throats.

Eucalyptus tea can be used to treat cold and flu symptoms and bronchitis, and to improve the immune system. The tea is made by steeping leaves in boiling water. You can also make a steam inhalation by boiling the leaves and breathing the steam to clear sinuses.

HOW TO GROW THIS PLANT

LIGHT: Direct sunlight is necessary.

WATER: Keep evenly moist during the summer growing season. In the winter, water when the top 1" of soil is dry.

TEMPERATURE: Keep in a slightly cool room.

TIPS: The tree will likely outgrow your available space within a few years. Before planting outside, check with your local extension office to see if it's considered invasive in your area.

Flamingo Lily

Anthurium andraeanum

DESCRIPTION

Dark green, heart-shaped leaves contrasting with deep red spathes and white or yellow flowers (spadices).

SIZE

Grows to a maximum of 2' tall, with leaves reaching 12" in length.

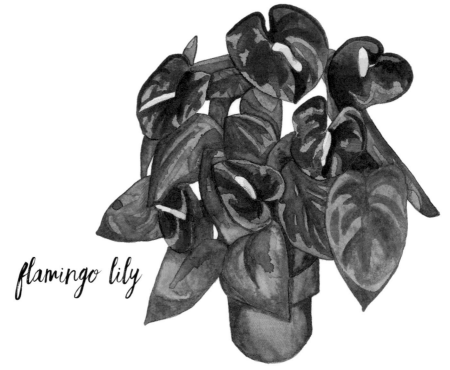

flamingo lily

❧ Removes airborne toxins   ❧ Increases daytime oxygen

The flamingo lily is a common decorative plant that does secret double duty as an air filter. These tropical aroids use their bright green, glossy leaves to remove industrial pollutants like xylene, formaldehyde, and ammonia from the indoor environment. Xylene, formaldehyde, and ammonia are found in manufactured goods such as furniture, and they aggravate the respiratory system and may increase the risk of cancer. Flamingo lilies are excellent when grouped with other air-purifying tropical plants, such as *Philodendron* species or the peace lily (a species of *Spathiphyllum*). Additionally, the more plants you have, the more oxygen they release into your home.

Be careful: you should never ingest any part of a flamingo lily, as it contains calcium oxalate crystals, which are a major irritant for soft tissues.

HOW TO GROW THIS PLANT

LIGHT: Bright, indirect sunlight is best; avoid direct sunlight.

WATER: Keep continuously moist and mist daily to maintain humidity. Leaf browning is a sign of low humidity or inadequate water.

TEMPERATURE: Keep in a warm, humid room, at a minimum of 70°F.

TIPS: A well-grown flamingo lily will flower intermittently all year, providing a virtually nonstop display of its striking spathe/spadix combination. Keep it slightly pot-bound for best results, and repot into a fresh peat-based soil mix annually.

Goethe Plant

Bryophyllum pinnatum (also *Kalanchoe pinnata*)

DESCRIPTION

Perennial succulents with fleshy, scallop-edged leaves on upright stalks. Bell-shaped, pale reddish flowers hang from stems.

SIZE

Can reach a maximum height of 18".

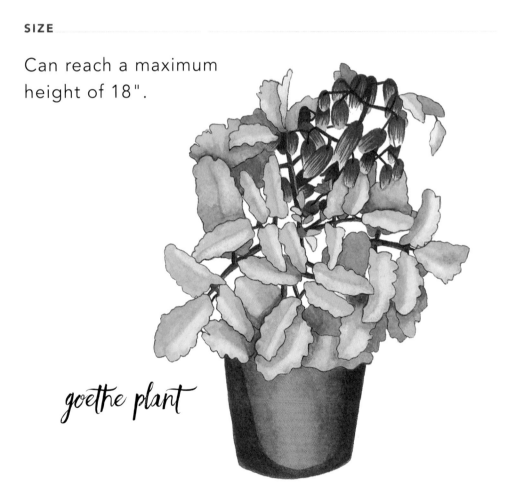

goethe plant

HEALTH BENEFITS

- Fights inflammation
- Promotes healthy skin
- Prevents kidney stones
- Fights gastric ulcers
- Promotes sleep
- Fights anxiety

Once treasured by famous writer Johann Wolfgang von Goethe, this perennial contains a range of health benefits. Oral extract of the Goethe plant is an effective anti-inflammatory. The extract is also used to treat kidney stones and fight the bacteria that cause stomach ulcers. It can also safely be consumed by expectant mothers as a sleep aid and to reduce anxiety.

To prepare the extract, remove and wash the leaves, then let them sit for five to seven days. Mince the leaves and press to remove the juice. Dissolve the juice in 20 percent ethanol and store in the refrigerator. To create a rub for treating skin irritations and wounds, mix the fresh-squeezed juice with lanolin. Consuming large quantities of the leaves may cause sickness in animals, so keep it out of reach of pets.

HOW TO GROW THIS PLANT

LIGHT: Bright, sunny windows or sunrooms are best.

WATER: Let soil surface dry between waterings; in the winter, water when the top 1" of soil is dry.

TEMPERATURE: Temperatures over 70°F are ideal.

TIPS: These hardy succulents are sometimes called the miracle plant because they produce plantlets along the leaf margins that can be potted to grow new plants.

Heartleaf Philodendron

Philodendron hederaceum (also *Philodendron cordatum*)

DESCRIPTION

Distinctive heart-shaped leaves on a climbing stem. Immature leaves are reddish bronze in color and deepen to green with time.

SIZE

Indoor stems are limited by support size and trimming. Leaves are a maximum of 5" long and up to 4" wide indoors.

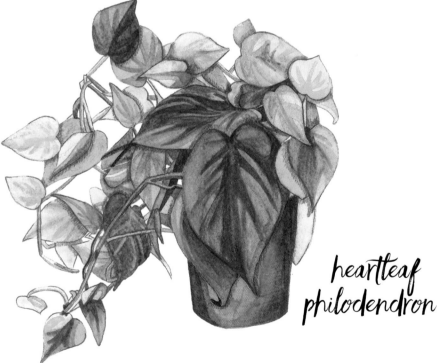

heartleaf philodendron

🍃 Removes airborne toxins   🍃 Increases daytime oxygen

Known as the heartleaf philodendron, the *P. hederaceum* is a tropical plant that is known for purifying indoor air. According to the University of Florida's Institute of Food and Agricultural Sciences, the heartleaf philodendron removes airborne formaldehyde, an industrial toxin (found in cleaning products and manufactured furniture) that causes respiratory distress. While the plant isn't distinguished by the volume of toxins it removes, it can survive better in low-light conditions than other indoor plants, making it a valuable addition to darker rooms. It also increases oxygen levels in your home through natural respiration.

Heartleaf philodendrons contain calcium oxalate crystals, which are an irritant, so avoid directly ingesting any part of the plant.

HOW TO GROW THIS PLANT

✴ **LIGHT:** Low to moderate light is ideal. Never expose to direct sunlight.

💧 **WATER:** Water weekly and mist leaves daily to maintain humidity.

⬤ **TEMPERATURE:** Warm temperatures above 70°F are ideal.

✳ **TIPS:** In its native environment, the plant climbs up trees by means of clinging roots. Indoors, however, it does best as a trailing plant or tied to a support. Trim growing tips to limit the size.

Hippeastrum

Hippeastrum species

DESCRIPTION

Large bulbs (up to 5") bloom into very large and showy funnel-shaped flowers in a variety of colors, with long, strap-like leaves.

SIZE

Flowers grow up to 8" across, with leaves 1" in width and up to 36" in length.

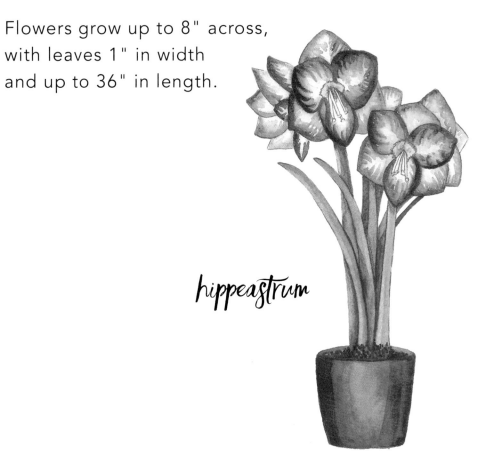

hippeastrum

HEALTH BENEFITS

- Promotes gastrointestinal health
- Fights viruses
- Fights inflammation

Because of its impressive flowers, many hybrids of the *Hippeastrum* genus have been created. The plant you want for its health benefits is the *H. puniceum*, a native of South America with orange flowers. Hippeastrum bulbs, which contain the alkaloid lycorine, are roasted or boiled and then used to make a tea that holistic medicine practitioners prescribe to treat stomachache. In small quantities, isolated lycorine has been shown to be antibacterial, antiviral, and anti-inflammatory. However, it's important to note that, at higher quantities, lycorine can cause vomiting and other serious symptoms.

HOW TO GROW THIS PLANT

LIGHT: Bright, filtered sunlight is ideal.

WATER: Bare bulbs should be planted in fresh peat and watered once to "wake up." Water weekly during the summer growing season, but never let sit in water. In the fall, as the leaves begin to die, withhold water to send the bulb back into dormancy.

TEMPERATURE: Room temperature is best.

TIPS: Once the yearly flowering is done, remove the dead flower stalks. When you have sent the bulb back into dormancy, it must remain dormant for two months in order to bloom again.

Holy Basil

Ocimum tenuiflorum (also *Ocimum sanctum*)

DESCRIPTION

Dark green, oval leaves that sometimes have a purplish cast.

SIZE

Can grow up to 3' tall.

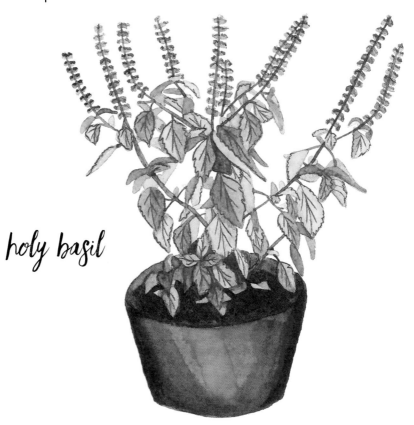

holy basil

- Fights bacterial infections
- Reduces cold and flu symptoms
- Promotes gastrointestinal health
- Fights inflammation
- Treats respiratory conditions
- Combats type 2 diabetes
- Improves blood sugar levels
- Fights heart disease and cancer
- Promotes healthy skin
- Reduces ear swelling and pain

From seeds to leaves to extracts, every part of holy basil—also called tulsi—is loaded with healing compounds. Tulsi essential oil has been shown to completely stop the growth of staph bacteria (including MRSA) and *E. coli*, both of which can cause dangerous illnesses.

The flowers and leaves of holy basil are used to treat coughs and colds; soothe upset stomach; reduce swelling and inflammation; and help treat conditions including type 2 diabetes, asthma, bronchitis, cancer, heart disease, diarrhea, and fever. The leaves can be chewed whole or crushed to extract the juice, which can be mixed into water. You can also use the leaf juice as an eardrop to help treat earaches and infection, or it can be applied directly to the skin to soothe insect bites.

HOW TO GROW THIS PLANT

LIGHT: Bright spots with several hours of direct sunlight are ideal.

WATER: Keep evenly moist.

TEMPERATURE: Normal room temperature is ideal.

TIPS: Pinch off growing tips and flower buds with a pair of sharp scissors or shears to encourage bushiness. You can harvest leaves as soon as the plant is established.

Hot Peppers

Cayenne, pequin, habanero, Thai, and other small, ornamental varieties

DESCRIPTION

Upright plants with oval, green leaves and clusters of peppers.

SIZE

Smaller than outdoor peppers, reaching 1"–1.5" in length on plants that are about 1' in height.

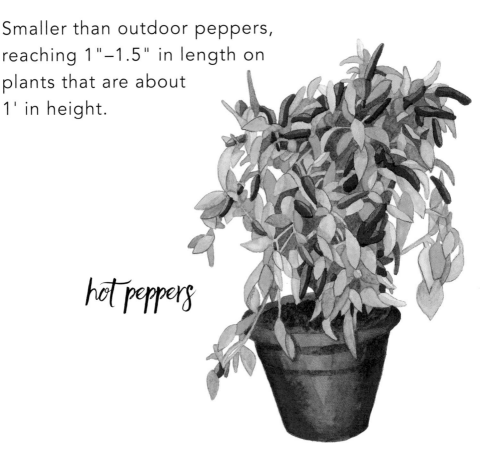

hot peppers

- Eases aches and pains
- Fights inflammation
- May promote weight loss
- Boosts immune system
- Lowers cholesterol
- Improves blood sugar levels
- Contains powerful antioxidants
- Contains vitamins

Hot or chili peppers have been an important part of the culinary tradition for thousands of years, and more recently scientists have discovered the health benefits of their main component, capsaicin. Capsaicin, the source of a pepper's heat, is a powerful metabolism booster and anti-inflammatory that is used to relieve pain and boost the immune system. It can also reduce cholesterol and aid in blood sugar management. Additionally, hot peppers are rich in antioxidants, vitamin A, vitamin D, and potassium. To get their health benefits, simply include the peppers in your favorite recipes (and get ready to sweat!).

HOW TO GROW THIS PLANT

LIGHT: Direct sunlight or bright artificial light is best. If you're starting from seed, use artificial light to get strong seedlings.

WATER: Keep evenly moist.

TEMPERATURE: Provide as much warmth during the day as possible, with cooler nights to encourage flowering.

TIPS: Fertilize established plants with a high-quality vegetable fertilizer, following the label directions. You can either buy young plants or start from seed indoors. Pinch off the first few flowers with a pair of sharp scissors or shears to encourage more pods.

Jasmine

Jasminum officinale

DESCRIPTION

Long, vining stems bear sets of leaves with five to nine leaflets and white, fragrant flowers.

SIZE

Vines can grow up to 30' tall outdoors. Indoors, you can prune them to fit your available space and support.

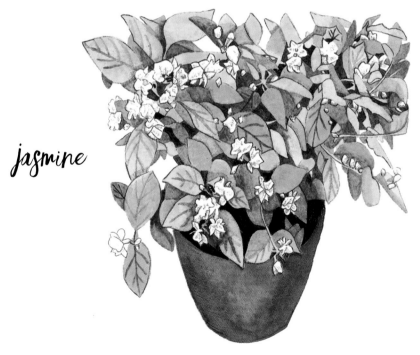

jasmine

- Eases aches and pains
- Fights anxiety
- Fights depression
- Works as an aphrodisiac
- Promotes healthy skin

Jasmine is popular in aromatherapy—but its healing properties go far beyond its lilting scent. Jasmine tea is used to treat headaches, anxiety, and depression, and it also acts as an aphrodisiac. To make jasmine tea, cut the flowers and mix them with loose tea leaves, then cover and let the flowers perfume the tea for at least twenty-four hours. Leave the flowers in the tea, and store in a cool, dry place.

You can also make an oil infusion by mixing jasmine flowers into a base oil such as extra-virgin olive oil. Seal and let it steep for up to forty-eight hours, then strain out the flowers. Jasmine oil can be applied directly to the skin to treat rash and irritation.

HOW TO GROW THIS PLANT

LIGHT: Bright, indirect sunlight is best.

WATER: Water weekly.

TEMPERATURE: Average room temperature is perfect, though it is tolerant of a wide range of temperatures.

TIPS: Jasmine needs a support such as a bark pole or wire frame to grow properly. When it starts to get too big, prune it back and use the cuttings to start a new plant. For medicinal use, make sure you're growing a true jasmine and not star jasmine, confederate jasmine, or other *Trachelospermum* species.

Kimberly Queen Fern

Nephrolepis obliterata

DESCRIPTION

Upright or drooping fronds with lightly scalloped leaflets.

SIZE

Can grow up to 3' tall.

kimberly queen fern

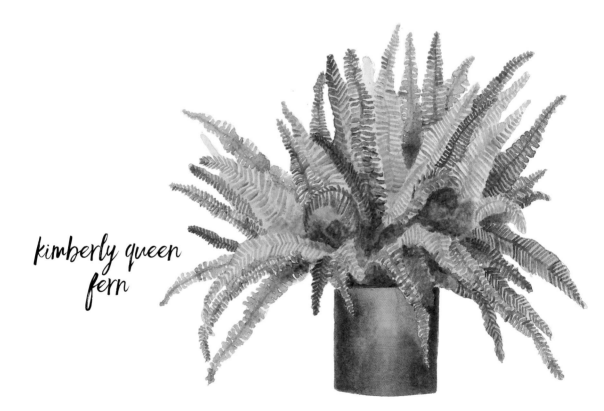

🌿 Removes airborne toxins   🌿 Increases daytime oxygen

The Kimberly Queen fern looks like an air filter—and for good reason: it is. This pretty fern has been studied by the renowned NASA researcher Dr. Bill Wolverton for its ability to remove toxins, including formaldehyde, toluene, and xylene, from indoor air. Toluene is a common industrial solvent used in paint, adhesives, glues, and other common household products. Breathing toluene fumes can make asthma worse. Formaldehyde and xylene are industrial by-products that can cause nausea, headaches, respiratory problems, and an increased risk of cancer. In his studies, Dr. Wolverton found that the Kimberly Queen fern wasn't as effective as the more popular Boston fern at removing formaldehyde from the air, but the plant makes up for this by being more tolerant of typical indoor conditions. It also increases oxygen levels through natural respiration.

HOW TO GROW THIS PLANT

LIGHT: Tolerant of a wide range of light conditions, from low light to bright, indirect sunlight.

WATER: Keep continuously moist; do not let dry out. Moderately drought tolerant.

TEMPERATURE: Room temperature is ideal. Avoid cold drafts.

TIPS: The Kimberly Queen fern is more compact and less messy than the Boston fern, making it an ideal candidate for indoor cultivation. During repotting, divide the root mass to easily propagate. These ferns are well suited to hanging containers.

Money Tree

Pachira aquatica

DESCRIPTION

A braided trunk, topped with lance-like, palmate leaves.

SIZE

While reaching 60' outdoors, indoor plant height depends on container size and pruning.

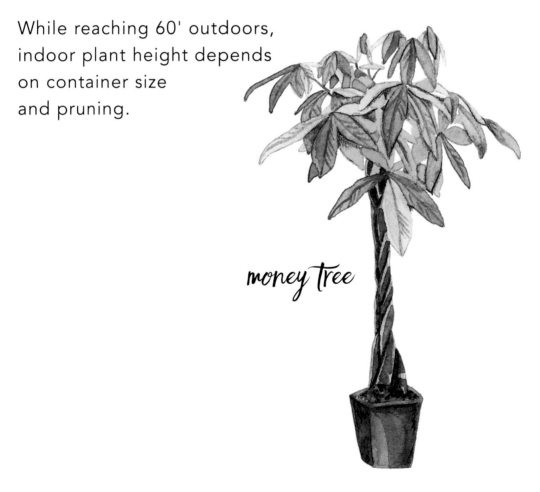

money tree

- Promotes healthy skin
- Eases aches and pains
- Promotes gastrointestinal health
- Removes airborne toxins

The braided money tree was introduced in the 1980s, when a Taiwanese truck driver braided several trunks together and discovered the plant would continue to grow. Today, these pretty braided trees are still used as feng shui objects, bringing good luck and prosperity.

A tonic made from soaking the bark in water overnight is used to treat headaches and stomach upset, while a poultice of the leaves is used to soothe minor skin irritation and burns. Additionally, a study conducted at the Hanyang University in South Korea found that the money tree removed toxins from indoor air. The plant was especially effective at removing benzene, along with xylene, formaldehyde, and toluene. These common industrial toxins are found in household cleaning products and furniture, and can cause respiratory issues and an increased risk of cancer.

HOW TO GROW THIS PLANT

LIGHT: Bright, indirect sunlight is best.

WATER: Water weekly, but let the soil dry between waterings. Mist leaves once daily or every few days to maintain humidity.

TEMPERATURE: A warm room is ideal.

TIPS: Money trees are hardy and not difficult to grow. It's common for new plants to shed some leaves as the tree adjusts.

Neem Tree

Azadirachta indica

DESCRIPTION

Long leaves with shiny, crinkled leaflets.

SIZE

Mature trees are 60' tall, but indoor plants are constrained by pot size. Mature leaves grow up to 12" in length.

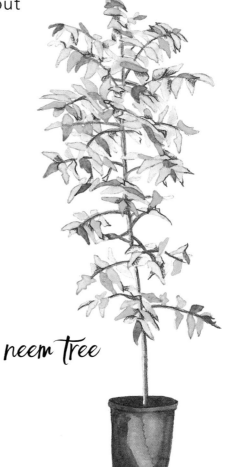

neem tree

HEALTH BENEFITS

- Fights inflammation
- Fights heart disease and cancer
- Improves blood sugar levels
- Fights infection
- Fights gastric ulcers
- Soothes itchy, red eyes
- Promotes oral hygiene

In India, neem has been an important component of the Ayurvedic medical system for centuries. A tea made from neem leaves fights inflammation, stomach ulcers, high blood sugar, bacterial and viral infections, heart disease, and cancer. To make the tea, simply boil the leaves in water and sweeten. A weak neem solution can be used to relieve red, itchy eyes, and powdered neem bark helps prevent gum disease. To make neem leaf extract, soak the leaves in water overnight, then grind the leaves in a container and strain the mixture. The longer you let the leaves steep, the stronger the mixture will be.

When using or preparing neem, be aware that at higher concentrations, neem can pose serious health risks. Always consult with a knowledgeable doctor or herbalist before consuming neem products.

HOW TO GROW THIS PLANT

LIGHT: Direct sunlight is preferred.

WATER: Water weekly, but let the soil dry between waterings.

TEMPERATURE: Warm temperatures are ideal.

TIPS: You'll likely be starting with a mail-order seed (neem is not a common nursery plant). To get the best results, fertilize weekly with a liquid fertilizer. You can harvest leaves once the plant is established.

Peace Lily

Spathiphyllum wallisii

DESCRIPTION

Deep green, lance-like, and upright leaves. The spadix is surrounded by a white spathe.

SIZE

Reaches up to 24" tall.

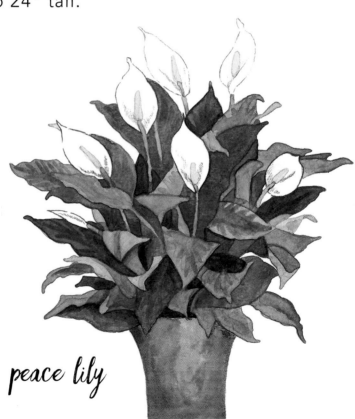

peace lily

HEALTH BENEFITS

🌿 Removes airborne toxins 🌿 Removes airborne mold

The peace lily is one of the most popular houseplants, thanks to its beauty and tolerance for low-light conditions. Fortunately, this plant is also a powerhouse when it comes to filtering air. In studies led by NASA researcher Dr. Bill Wolverton, the peace lily effectively filtered benzene, formaldehyde, trichloroethylene (TCE), xylene, toluene, and ammonia from indoor air. These industrial toxins are found in cleaning products and furniture, and can cause headaches, respiratory problems, and an increased risk of cancer.

According to other studies, the peace lily is also capable of removing airborne mold, which can help to alleviate allergies and asthma symptoms. Place a few plants in your bathroom to help reduce mold growth.

Be careful not to consume the leaves directly, as they contain calcium oxalate, which is an irritant for people and animals.

HOW TO GROW THIS PLANT

☀ **LIGHT:** Filtered sunlight is preferred.

💧 **WATER:** Water weekly and mist the leaves daily. Reduce water in winter and water only when the top 1" of soil is dry.

⬤ **TEMPERATURE:** Provide humid warmth and avoid cold drafts. Brown leaves are a sign of cold drafts or low humidity.

✳ **TIPS:** Peace lilies grow well in the same container for a year or more. Only repot when the soil is exhausted or the roots have formed a mass.

Phalaenopsis

Phalaenopsis species

DESCRIPTION

Large, green, paddle-shaped leaves on a single stem. Flower spikes bear clusters of large, round flowers.

SIZE

Plants reach a maximum height of 1', with flower spikes that grow to 2' tall.

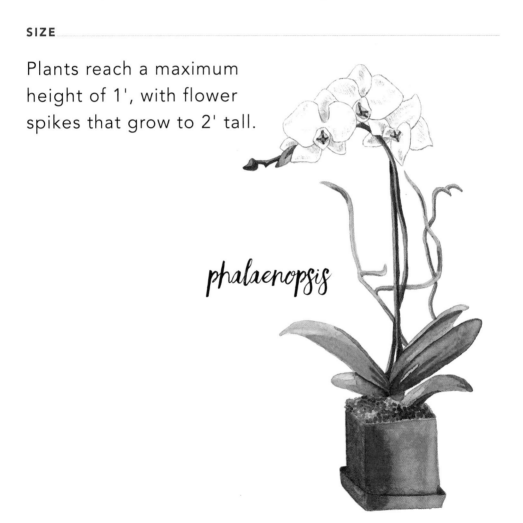

phalaenopsis

HEALTH BENEFITS

🌿 Removes airborne toxins   🌿 Increases daytime oxygen

The phalaenopsis orchid (also known as the moth orchid) is relatively slow-growing and doesn't have tremendous leaf surface area, which makes it a bit of a surprise that it is an air purifier. Still, in his studies on commonly grown indoor plants, NASA researcher Dr. Bill Wolverton found that phalaenopsis orchids filter formaldehyde from indoor air. Formaldehyde is an industrial toxin found in a number of manufactured goods and household cleaners; this toxin can lead to issues such as trouble breathing and headaches.

This beautiful orchid also increases oxygen levels in your home.

HOW TO GROW THIS PLANT

LIGHT: Provide bright, filtered sunlight.

WATER: Water regularly during the summer growing season. Reduce watering to twice per week during the winter. Never let water sit in the central junction where the leaves join the stem.

TEMPERATURE: Temperatures higher than 70°F during the summer growing season are preferred. In the fall, provide a week or two of 50°F nighttime temperatures to stimulate flowering.

TIPS: After flowering, cut off the dead flower spike at the base and move to a bright windowsill. The plant may bloom again the following year.

Pothos Vine

Epipremnum aureum (also *Scindapsus aureus*)

DESCRIPTION

Fast-growing vine with heart-shaped leaves.

SIZE

Vines can grow in excess of 50', but indoor plants
can easily be pruned to fit your space.
Leaves range from 2" long up to 12" long
on mature plants.

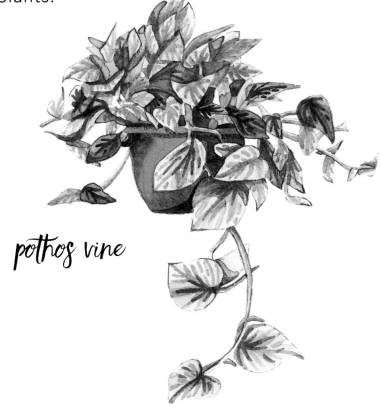

pothos vine

HEALTH BENEFITS

🍃 Removes airborne toxins   🍃 Increases daytime oxygen

Pothos vines (a.k.a. Devil's Ivy) are notoriously tough, as they will survive for a long time in challenging growing environments (e.g. poor light and uneven watering). At the same time, the beautiful green and yellow leaves excel at filtering out the industrial toxins benzene, formaldehyde, xylene, and toluene from indoor air. These harmful toxins are found in a number of manufactured goods and can cause respiratory issues and an increased risk of cancer. Thanks to its fast metabolism, the pothos vine also increases indoor oxygen levels. No part of this plant should be consumed by people or animals, however, as it contains a mild toxin that can cause stomach upset.

HOW TO GROW THIS PLANT

☀ **LIGHT:** Moderate to bright light is preferred.

💧 **WATER:** Keep soil moist.

⬤ **TEMPERATURE:** Warm rooms are ideal.

✳ **TIPS:** Pothos can be grown up a support, as a trailing plant, or as a hanging vine. Cuttings easily propagate in water. To start a new plant, take a piece of the vine, remove the bottom two or three sets of leaves, and set the cutting in a cup of water. Keep the water fresh. When new roots emerge, pot into a new container with soil.

Rosemary

Rosmarinus officinalis

DESCRIPTION

Evergreen shrub with pointed leaves that look like pine needles.

SIZE

Can grow up to 2' tall. Leaves reach 1" in length.

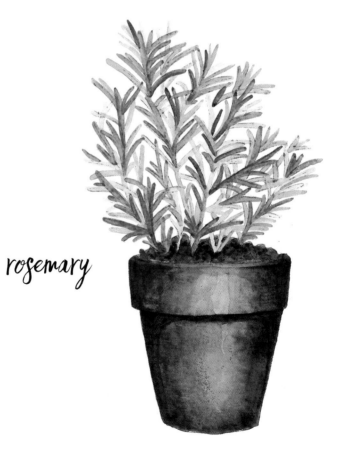

rosemary

HEALTH BENEFITS

- Contains powerful antioxidants
- Promotes brain health
- Fights heart disease and cancer
- Treats dyspepsia
- Promotes healthy hair
- Eases aches and pains
- Reduces stress
- Antimicrobial

The leaves of this fragrant herb are packed with antioxidants, including carnosic acid and rosmarinic acid. Consuming rosemary has been shown to improve memory and brain function and fight heart disease. Rosemary is also approved by the German Commission E for the treatment of dyspepsia. Rosemary oil, which is commonly available in health stores, is a popular topical treatment for muscle pain, and studies have shown that rubbing rosemary oil into the scalp can help prevent alopecia (hair loss). Rosemary has also shown antimicrobial activity, and may inhibit the growth of tumors.

When used in aromatherapy, rosemary reduces stress. Try placing sachets of rosemary in different rooms to enjoy the wonderful fragrance and its calming effects.

HOW TO GROW THIS PLANT

LIGHT: Strong sunlight is ideal. Place in front of a south-facing window if possible. If your plants aren't growing well, try adding artificial lights; the most common problem with indoor rosemary is insufficient light.

WATER: Thoroughly water when dry, then let drain completely.

TEMPERATURE: Room temperature is best; avoid humid conditions.

TIPS: Rosemary can be susceptible to powdery mildew when grown inside. Look for a slightly fluffy white powder on the leaves. Remove affected leaves immediately.

Rubber Plant

Ficus elastica

DESCRIPTION

Large, oval, green leaves with a prominent central rib. Aerial roots develop on the trunks of larger specimens.

SIZE

Grows to 80' outdoors. Indoor plants are limited by container size and pruning.

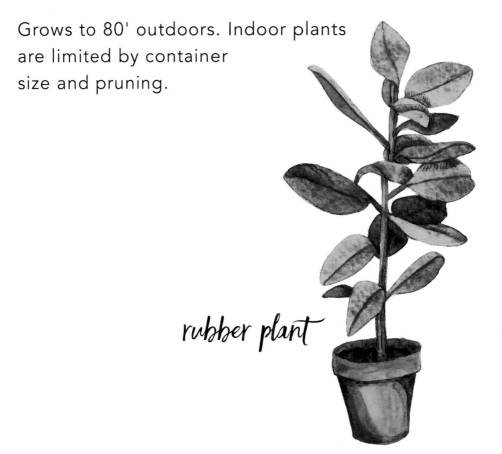

rubber plant

❧ Removes airborne toxins   ❧ Fights parasitic diseases

Ficus elastica earned the name rubber plant thanks to its sticky white latex, which was once used to make rubber. Today, it is a widely planted ornamental tree throughout the tropics. Indoors, the plant's very large, decorative leaves serve another purpose: helping purify the air. The rubber plant was shown in lab studies to be effective at removing formaldehyde, an industrial toxin found in cleaning supplies and furniture that causes respiratory problems.

Researchers are also studying compounds extracted from the rubber plant to combat tropical diseases and parasites. However, the sap of this plant is a mild irritant, so do not consume the plant or handle the sap with bare hands.

HOW TO GROW THIS PLANT

LIGHT: Bright, indirect sunlight is ideal, though it can tolerate low-light conditions.

WATER: Keep continuously moist but not soggy.

TEMPERATURE: Average room temperature is best.

TIPS: Occasionally wipe the leaves with a moist cloth or paper towel to keep their pores open for optimal air purification. When your rubber plant reaches the maximum allowed height, pinch off the growing tips with a pair of sharp scissors or shears to encourage side shoots. Repot large plants every other year, or when they are root-bound.

Sage

Salvia officinalis

DESCRIPTION

Perennial herb with gray-green, oval leaves.

SIZE

Reaches up to 2' tall.

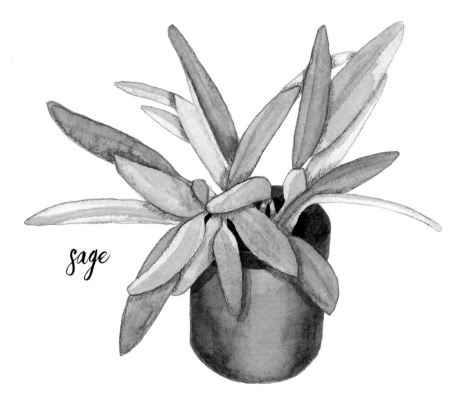

sage

HEALTH BENEFITS

- Contains powerful antioxidants
- Antibacterial
- Fights inflammation
- Promotes brain health
- Fights depression
- Lowers cholesterol
- May promote weight loss
- Combats type 2 diabetes
- Reduces hot flashes
- Promotes gastrointestinal health

One of the oldest medicinal plants in the world, sage contains powerful antioxidants, antibacterials, and anti-inflammatories.

A tea made by steeping the leaves in hot water for five minutes helps fight type 2 diabetes, while leaves consumed raw treat hot flashes. Sage extracts and oil have been shown to improve memory and mood, help manage Alzheimer's disease, lower cholesterol, suppress appetite, and fight cancer. To make an oil infusion, place crushed leaves in a jar of oil (such as olive oil), let the mixture sit for forty-eight hours, and then strain out the leaves. The oil can then be directly consumed. Sage leaves, tea, and extract are also excellent at soothing stomach pain and can help reduce symptoms associated with irritable bowel syndrome.

HOW TO GROW THIS PLANT

LIGHT: Direct sunlight is needed. If you can't provide at least five hours of direct sunlight daily, use artificial lights.

WATER: Water weekly, but don't soak.

TEMPERATURE: Average room temperature is ideal.

TIPS: Sage propagates easily from cuttings. To start a new plant, remove the top section of a branch and trim off the lowest leaves, but leave at least three sets of leaves intact. Insert the cutting into soil, and keep it warm and moist until new growth starts.

Selloum Philodendron

Philodendron bipinnatifidum

DESCRIPTION

Large aroid with deeply lobed leaves.

SIZE

Can grow up to 5', with leaves reaching 3' in length.

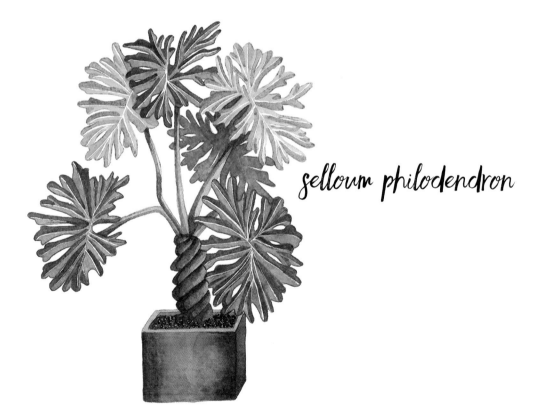

selloum philodendron

HEALTH BENEFITS

ℰ᷎ Removes airborne toxins   ℰ᷎ Increases daytime oxygen

It's easy to imagine the giant leaves of this gorgeous tropical plant sucking pollutants from the air—which is exactly what it does. Researchers at Colorado State University and the University of Florida found that it is most effective at removing formaldehyde, a common toxin found in household cleaners and furniture that causes respiratory problems and may increase your risk of cancer.

The selloum philodendron also increases oxygen levels in your home during the day, creating even more clean, breathable air. Like other philodendrons, no part of this plant should be consumed directly by people or animals, as it contains an irritant that can cause stomach upset.

HOW TO GROW THIS PLANT

LIGHT: Indirect or dappled bright sunlight is best. It is tolerant of lower light but will grow more slowly.

WATER: Water weekly and mist daily to maintain humidity.

TEMPERATURE: Average to warm temperatures are best.

TIPS: This philodendron does not climb but slowly grows from a central trunk that sends out occasional aerial roots. For best results, keep it slightly pot-bound and push the aerial roots back into the potting soil. Fertilize at the beginning of the summer growing season with a controlled-release fertilizer. Be careful to follow label instructions.

Snake Plant

Sansevieria trifasciata

DESCRIPTION

Erect, spear-like, and stiff leaves, often with yellow or green coloration.

SIZE

Individual leaves may be greater than 2' long.

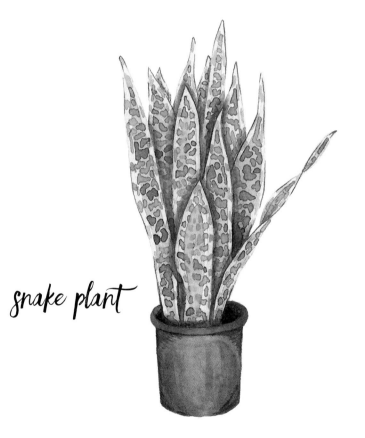

snake plant

HEALTH BENEFITS

- Removes airborne toxins
- Promotes healthy skin
- Eases aches and pains

Used as a houseplant in the United States for the last century, the snake plant is one of the most recognizable indoor plants in the country. It is effective at removing a wide variety of airborne pollutants, including benzene, formaldehyde, trichloroethylene (TCE), xylene, and toluene. These toxins are found in many manufactured goods and cleaning products and can result in respiratory ailments, headaches, and an increased risk of cancer.

The snake plant is also used in holistic medicine as a pain reliever and to treat skin irritation. The leaves are boiled to create a weak solution that can be applied directly to the skin. This plant should not be consumed by people or animals, however, as it contains saponin, a chemical that can cause gastrointestinal upset.

HOW TO GROW THIS PLANT

LIGHT: Bright light is best, but it is tolerant of a wide range of light conditions.

WATER: Water when the top 1" of soil is dry. Never let sit in water.

TEMPERATURE: Can adapt to both cool and warm temperatures.

TIPS: These are tough, striking plants that are easy to grow. If individual spears become loose in the potting soil, repot and pack fresh potting soil around the roots.

South African Geranium

Pelargonium sidoides

DESCRIPTION

Gray, felted leaves with ruffled edges and red wine or burgundy colored flowers.

SIZE

Grows up to 2' tall indoors.

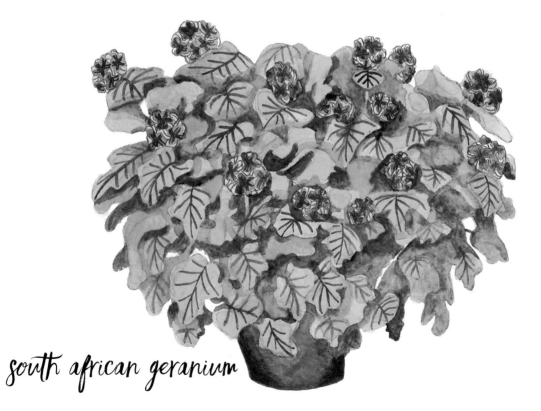

south african geranium

HEALTH BENEFITS

- ~ Promotes gastrointestinal health
- ~ Treats respiratory conditions
- ~ Reduces cold and flu symptoms

Native to Africa, the *P. sidoides* is a popular medicinal plant with an impressive array of health benefits. The main medicinal part of the plant is the root, which contains powerful polyphenols, proteins, and other compounds that have been shown to interfere with the ability of microbes to bind to host cells. In holistic medicine, it's used to treat stomach ailments and diarrhea, along with respiratory infections including the common cold, bronchitis, and strep throat. You can make your own extract by steeping powdered root in boiling water, then straining until it's clear. Take the extract directly or add to soothing teas.

HOW TO GROW THIS PLANT

LIGHT: Bright light is best. Provide at least four hours of direct sunlight.

WATER: Moderately drought tolerant. Water weekly and never let sit in water.

TEMPERATURE: Warm rooms are ideal.

TIPS: The South African geranium is perfect for growing in containers, providing you can give it enough light. During the summer growing season, provide with weekly liquid fertilizer. If you're planning to harvest the root, let the plant grow for at least one year before digging up and harvesting (although some sources say the roots are most potent after three years).

Spearmint

Mentha spicata (also *Mentha viridis*)

DESCRIPTION

Perennial herb bearing lance-shaped, finely serrated leaves on upright stems.

SIZE

Can reach 2' in height.

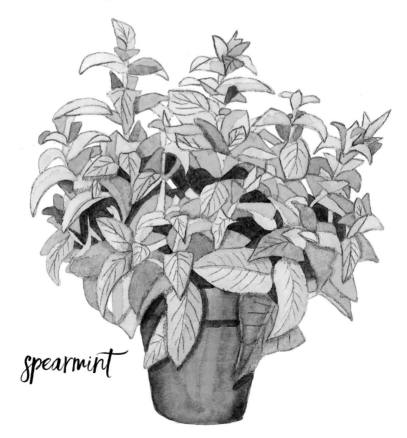

spearmint

- Promotes oral hygiene
- Fights inflammation
- Reduces cold and flu symptoms
- Fights anxiety
- Reduces stress
- Promotes gastrointestinal health
- Antibacterial

Common mint, or spearmint, has been used as a medicinal plant since ancient Rome, where it was a disinfectant, deodorant, and remedy for stomachaches. Fortunately for the ancients, there is sound science behind spearmint. The plant's leaves are rich in carvone, limonene, and menthol, all of which have been extensively studied for their health benefits.

Chewing spearmint leaves helps fight bad breath and oral infections. Tea brewed from spearmint leaves is used as an anti-inflammatory that can help soothe sore throats and chest congestion, as well as reduce anxiety and stress. Pregnant women also love spearmint tea because it helps fend off morning sickness and nausea. To make spearmint tea, steep fresh leaves in warm water for five minutes, then sweeten with a natural sweetener.

HOW TO GROW THIS PLANT

LIGHT: Direct sunlight is preferred.

WATER: Keep evenly moist.

TEMPERATURE: Temperatures over 65°F are ideal.

TIPS: All varieties of mint are aggressive growers, so avoid planting multiple types in the same pot. Mint starts easily from seed. You can begin to harvest leaves as soon as the plant is established. Pinch off flower buds with a pair of sharp scissors or shears to extend its useful life.

Spider Plant

Chlorophytum comosum

DESCRIPTION

Narrow, typically striped leaves that form clumps. Plantlets emerge on long, trailing shoots.

SIZE

Leaves can reach 12", with hanging shoots reaching 18".

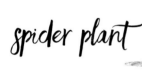

spider plant

- Removes airborne toxins
- Traps and removes particulate matter

The spider plant is named for the look of its hanging plantlets, which resemble baby spiders hanging on strands of web beneath the mother plant. In air quality studies, the spider plant was shown to filter out formaldehyde, xylene, benzene, and toluene from indoor air. In a study published in *Plant Physiology and Biochemistry* in 2017, the spider plant was identified as the most "efficient benzene removal plant" among all the plants screened. Formaldehyde, xylene, benzene, and toluene are commonly used in solvents and manufacturing, and they are known to cause respiratory problems and headaches, and may even increase your risk of cancer.

In a study published in *Air Quality, Atmosphere and Health*, scientists tested the spider plant for its ability to remove "particulate matter" (dust, mold, and smoke) from indoor environments. They found that spider plants are excellent at removing these dangerous pollutants by trapping them in leaf wax.

HOW TO GROW THIS PLANT

LIGHT: Medium to bright light is needed.

WATER: Water weekly and mist daily. Hanging plants tend to dry out faster, so be sure to keep up with watering.

TEMPERATURE: Average room temperature is best.

TIPS: Use a liquid fertilizer with every watering during the summer growing season. Remove and pot individual plantlets to easily propagate.

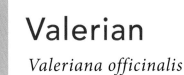

Valerian

Valeriana officinalis

DESCRIPTION

Clusters of pink or white flowers suspended on compound leaves.

SIZE

Grows up to 5' outside but can be maintained at 2'–3' indoors.

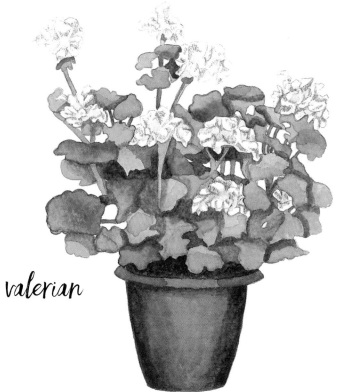

valerian

HEALTH BENEFITS

🌿 Reduces stress 🌿 Reduces PMS symptoms

🌿 Promotes sleep

Valerian, nicknamed "heal all" in the Middle Ages, is loaded with health-promoting components. Valerian leaves and roots promote healthy sleep and calm jittery nerves. In one recent study, valerian root extract was shown to reduce the symptoms of premenstrual syndrome.

Make a decoction from the grated root by gently boiling it in water, then straining the mixture. Consume it as a calming tea. You can also make a valerian tincture by soaking valerian root in alcohol (typically vodka) for up to five weeks. Strain the root out and store the resulting tincture in a cool, dark place. To use the tincture as a sleep aid, start with ¼ teaspoon at first, taken before bed.

HOW TO GROW THIS PLANT

☀ **LIGHT:** Provide as much direct sunlight as possible, or use artificial lights.

💧 **WATER:** Water weekly.

⬤ **TEMPERATURE:** Average room temperature is preferred, though it can tolerate temperatures down to 50°F.

✳ **TIPS:** Start your valerian from seed, then transplant. It will bloom in late spring or early summer. To harvest the roots, dig up mature plants (at least one year old), clean the roots, then snip roots into 1" sections. Allow the roots to air-dry for three weeks. The drying roots emit a strong odor that attracts cats, so find a safe place to dry your roots!

Weeping Fig

Ficus benjamina

DESCRIPTION

Glossy, oval leaves on a smooth trunk.

SIZE

Can reach 100' tall in its native habitat. Indoor size is constrained by container and pruning.

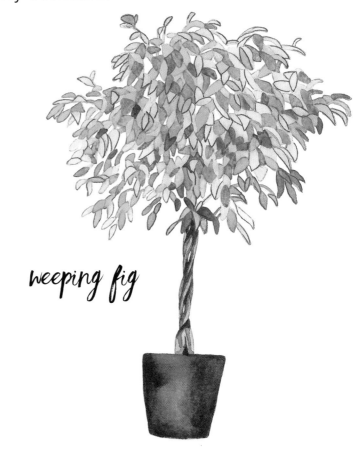

weeping fig

HEALTH BENEFITS

✿ Removes airborne toxins   ✿ Fights viruses

The weeping fig is a popular and beautiful interior plant that filters some of the more common household toxins from the air, including formaldehyde, benzene, trichloroethylene (TCE), xylene, and toluene. Of all the pollutants tested, it was most effective against formaldehyde, filtering out almost 50 percent of the chemical in a laboratory study. These toxins are found in furniture and household cleaners and can cause respiratory problems and headaches.

Scientists are also discovering new medicinal uses for this beautiful tree. One group of researchers at Ben-Gurion University of the Negev in Israel found that a tincture of weeping fig strongly inhibited the herpes virus. However, any use of extracts from this plant should be approached with caution. The sap of the weeping fig is an irritant and can result in skin and respiratory irritation.

HOW TO GROW THIS PLANT

☀ **LIGHT:** Bright, indirect sunlight is preferred.

💧 **WATER:** Keep moist, but don't let sit in water.

● **TEMPERATURE:** Average room temperatures are ideal. Dropping leaves may be a sign of cold drafts.

✳ **TIPS:** Indoors, keep this fast-growing tree under control through a combination of carefully timed repotting and trimming. Repot younger plants annually and older plants every other year or so. When pruning, remove lower branches first. Moving the plant too frequently can result in leaf drop.

ZZ Plant

Zamioculcas zamiifolia

DESCRIPTION

Evergreen aroid with oval leaflets borne on leaves that emerge directly from an underground rhizome.

SIZE

Can grow up to 3' tall.

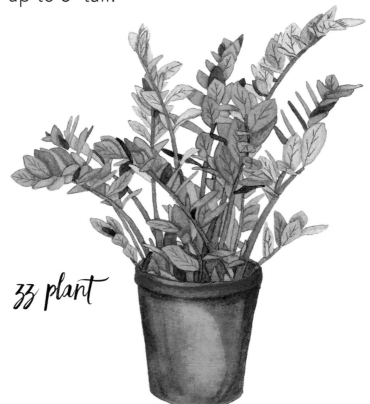

zz plant

❧ Removes airborne toxins   ❧ Increases daytime oxygen

This common houseplant improves indoor air quality by removing benzene, toluene, and xylene—toxins that contribute to "sick building syndrome," a collection of symptoms that includes frequent headaches, dizziness, respiratory problems, allergies, asthma, and other issues connected to chronic exposure to indoor pollutants.

According to an experiment conducted at the King Mongkut's University of Technology in Bangkok, the ZZ plant was the best plant for removing xylene from indoor air. Better yet, the ZZ plant continues purifying the air even when it isn't getting adequate water or light, while also increasing oxygen levels in your home. The sap of this plant is an irritant, so be careful when directly handling the leaves, and no part of the ZZ plant should be consumed by people or animals.

HOW TO GROW THIS PLANT

LIGHT: Adapts easily to a wide range of conditions, from low light to bright, indirect sunlight.

WATER: Water when the top 1" of soil is dry. Do not overwater or let sit in water. Brown leaves may be a sign of overwatering. Mist daily to increase humidity.

TEMPERATURE: Average room temperature is ideal. Low humidity may cause leaves to brown.

TIPS: Fertilize with a high-quality, controlled-release fertilizer at the beginning of the summer growing season. Follow the label directions.

Appendix: Houseplants by Health Benefit

Looking for which plants can help soothe a sunburn or calm an upset stomach? The following appendix makes it easy to search for plants by their health benefits.

ANTIBACTERIAL

- Basil
- Eucalyptus
- Sage
- Spearmint

ANTIMICROBIAL

- Basil
- Rosemary

AROMATHERAPEUTIC

- Dwarf French lavender

BOOSTS IMMUNE SYSTEM

- Dendrobium
- Eucalyptus
- Hot peppers

COMBATS TYPE 2 DIABETES

- Aloe vera
- Banana
- Holy basil
- Sage

CONTAINS POWERFUL ANTIOXIDANTS

- Aloe vera
- Basil
- Crocus
- Hot peppers
- Rosemary
- Sage

CONTAINS VITAMINS

- Hot peppers

EASES ACHES AND PAINS

- Avocado
- Hot peppers
- Jasmine
- Money tree
- Rosemary
- Snake plant

FIGHTS ANXIETY

- Goethe plant
- Jasmine
- Spearmint

FIGHTS BACTERIAL INFECTIONS

- Aloe vera
- Holy basil

FIGHTS DEPRESSION

- Basil
- Jasmine
- Sage

FIGHTS GASTRIC ULCERS

- Aloe vera
- Banana
- Goethe plant
- Neem tree

FIGHTS HEART DISEASE AND CANCER

- Aloe vera
- Crocus
- Holy basil
- Neem tree
- Rosemary

FIGHTS INFECTION

- Neem tree

FIGHTS INFLAMMATION

- Aloe vera
- Basil
- English ivy
- Goethe plant
- Hippeastrum
- Holy basil
- Hot peppers
- Neem tree
- Sage
- Spearmint

FIGHTS PARASITIC DISEASES

- Rubber plant

FIGHTS VIRUSES

- Hippeastrum
- Weeping fig

IMPROVES BLOOD SUGAR LEVELS

- Avocado
- Dendrobium
- Holy basil
- Hot peppers
- Neem tree

INCREASES DAYTIME OXYGEN

- Bromeliads
- Chinese evergreen
- Chocolate oncidium
- *Dracaena deremensis* 'Janet Craig'
- *Dracaena deremensis* 'Warneckii'

INCREASES DAYTIME OXYGEN—*CONTINUED*

- *Dracaena fragrans* 'Massangeana'
- *Dracaena marginata*
- Dumb cane
- Dwarf date palm
- Emerald Gem
- English ivy
- Flamingo lily
- Heartleaf philodendron
- Kimberly Queen fern
- Phalaenopsis
- Pothos vine
- Selloum philodendron
- ZZ plant

INCREASES HUMIDITY

- Bamboo palm
- Boston fern

INCREASES NIGHTTIME OXYGEN

- Barberton daisy
- Christmas cactus

LOWERS CHOLESTEROL

- Avocado
- Hot peppers
- Sage

MAY PROMOTE WEIGHT LOSS

- Areca palm
- Avocado
- Dendrobium
- Hot peppers
- Sage

PREVENTS KIDNEY STONES

- Goethe plant

PROMOTES BRAIN HEALTH

- Avocado
- Dendrobium
- Rosemary
- Sage

PROMOTES GASTROINTESTINAL HEALTH

- Aloe vera
- Basil
- Chinese jade plant
- Dendrobium
- Hippeastrum
- Holy basil
- Money tree
- Sage
- South African geranium
- Spearmint

PROMOTES HEALTHY HAIR

- Aloe vera
- Rosemary

PROMOTES HEALTHY SKIN

- Aloe vera
- Avocado
- Banana
- Chinese jade plant
- Eucalyptus
- Goethe plant
- Holy basil
- Jasmine
- Money tree
- Snake plant

PROMOTES ORAL HYGIENE

- Aloe vera
- Neem tree
- Spearmint

PROMOTES SLEEP

- Crocus
- Dwarf French lavender
- Goethe plant
- Valerian

REDUCES COLD AND FLU SYMPTOMS

- Banana
- Eucalyptus
- Holy basil
- South African geranium
- Spearmint

REDUCES EAR SWELLING AND PAIN

- Holy basil

REDUCES HOT FLASHES

- Sage

REDUCES PMS SYMPTOMS

- Crocus
- Valerian

REDUCES STRESS

- Basil
- Dwarf French lavender
- Rosemary
- Spearmint
- Valerian

REMOVES AIRBORNE MOLD

- Peace lily

REMOVES AIRBORNE TOXINS

- Areca palm
- Bamboo palm
- Barberton daisy
- Boston fern
- Bromeliads
- Chinese evergreen
- Chocolate oncidium
- Christmas cactus
- *Dracaena deremensis* 'Janet Craig'
- *Dracaena deremensis* 'Warneckii'
- *Dracaena fragrans* 'Massangeana'
- *Dracaena marginata*
- Dumb cane
- Dwarf date palm
- Elephant ear philodendron
- Emerald Gem
- English ivy
- Flamingo lily
- Heartleaf philodendron
- Kimberly Queen fern
- Money tree

REMOVES AIRBORNE TOXINS—*CONTINUED*

- Peace lily
- Phalaenopsis
- Pothos vine
- Rubber plant
- Selloum philodendron
- Snake plant
- Spider plant
- Weeping fig
- ZZ plant

REMOVES HYDROCARBONS

- Elephant ear philodendron

SOOTHES ITCHY, RED EYES

- Neem tree

TRAPS AND REMOVES PARTICULATE MATTER

- Spider plant

TREATS DYSPEPSIA

- Rosemary

TREATS RESPIRATORY CONDITIONS

- Banana
- Crocus
- English ivy
- Eucalyptus
- Holy basil
- South African geranium

WORKS AS AN APHRODISIAC

- Jasmine

About the Author

Master gardener Jon VanZile's articles on gardening have appeared in the *Chicago Tribune*, *Better Homes and Gardens* special interest publications, the *Sun-Sentinel* (Ft. Lauderdale), the *Orlando Sentinel*, and other outlets. He was the houseplants and indoor gardening expert at About.com (now TheSpruce.com) for almost a decade, and made weekly guest expert appearances as the "garden guru" on the WSFL-TV morning show for several years.